"Dear Mrs. Carter,

I last had contact with you when you wrote me about taking your teachings to the Third World countries for missionaries. Well, I recently returned from Jamaica on just such a trip. I had great success. When coupled with fasting and prayer, the health was improved tremendously by just one treatment, and I was able to teach a pastor, his wife, and two townspeople to apply the method. We taped the training for future review, and I intend to return to teach large classes at a later date.

My hands have become very sensitive to the touch of people where I can feel their hurts, and my body remains in a state of extreme heat that is felt by the client as I work on them. My husband says he can feel an energy exchange just by being close to me, and I wondered if you experience this too. The doctors that have let me work on them stated that I was a more accurate diagnostician than they were and that most of the time that was a threat to the medical society that makes tons of insurance money when modern medicine is practiced but in Third World situations any medicine is welcomed. Please let me hear from you when you have the chance."

—B.V., Florida

"Dear Mrs. Carter,

You have done what I have long wished I had the time to do: a book on reflexology and nutrition combined. I have said that reflexology is just as good as the bloodstream; stimulating the circulation doesn't help much unless the blood is rich with nutrients that heal, and clean.

For many years I had a very painful condition almost half way up my back, to the right and under the ribs. Doctors invariably sent me for X-rays, and shrugged their shoulders: "There's nothing wrong with your lungs." Somewhere I read that such pain was from the liver, but still had no remedy. I decided to try reflexology—I couldn't feel many sore buttons anywhere, hands or feet, but often felt better after general treatment. One day I found what felt like a boil under my skin. It was under the little toe and the one next to it, down a little, like into the root of the little toe of the right foot, with no soreness on the left foot. I rubbed it out; the pain completely left my back area described above! A few times since, it has recurred, but a short treatment cures it again. I wanted to share this with others who suffer with frustration and no cure. I don't believe I have found this in other books. I also treat the inside, back, and front of my toes on left foot, which helps my hearing.

Sincerely,"

—W.P., Canada

"Dear Ms. Carter,

It is now just over twelve months since I came to you and told you that doctors at Gardner Hospital told me that I had leukemia and that my life span was probably from twelve to eighteen months. You know how I felt at that time and just how difficult it was to accept those facts. Since that time, I have made considerable progress, and it is now with immense satisfaction that I am able to advise you that due to progress made, my doctors are now planning on five-year life cycles for me, and at the present time, I am in complete remission.

To what my doctors may feel is due to medical progress, I feel that in the main, I have two very significant factors to which I am now able to contribute to my progress. One is the volumes of prayers which my friends have said on my behalf, and the other is the support which you have given me, both mentally and actually, by the volume of time you have given me with reflexology.

You will, doubtless, recall that when you first commenced on my hands, the results seemed infinitesimal, and that, at first, my feet were so tender that I could not wear my shoes nor could I bear for you to touch them. But, now, I am able to wear shoes and the results of my blood test continually show that my organs are now coping on their own.

It has now been three months since I have had regular reflexology, relying only on the reflexology treatments from you. Words cannot say thanks enough for giving me a new life span. You may feel at times that I am not appreciative for what you have done for me. The fact that I am now able to resume a normal forty-hour job will, I am sure, give you immense satisfaction. All I can say is, thank you for all that you have done for me. Not only for myself but for those that love me.

My doctors also share in my amazement at the progress I have made. Thank God for you and reflexology.

Sincerely,"

—A.K., Australia

BODY
Reflexology
REVISED & UPDATED EDITION

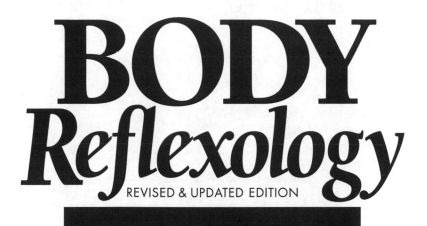

HEALING AT YOUR FINGERTIPS

MILDRED CARTER
& TAMMY WEBER

PARKER PUBLISHING COMPANY
West Nyack, New York 10995

Photographs by:
Jennifer Rodgers

10 9 8 7 6 5 4 3 2 1

This book is a reference work based on research by the author. Any techniques and suggestions are to be used at the reader's sole discretion. The
opinions expressed herein are not necessarily those of or endorsed by the
publisher. The directions stated in this book are in no way to be considered as a substitute for consultation with a duly licensed doctor.

Library of Congress Cataloging-in-Publication Data

Carter, Mildred.
   Body reflexology : healing at your fingertips / Mildred Carter &
Tammy Weber ; photographs by Jennifer Rodgers. — Rev. ed.
       p.   cm.
   Originally published: New York : Parker Pub. Co., 1983.
   Includes index.
   ISBN 0–13–299728–2.   ISBN 0–13–299736–3
   1. Reflexotherapy.   I. Weber, Tammy.   II. Title.
RM723.R43C37   1994
615.8'22—dc20   94–15863
                                               CIP

ISBN 0-13-299728-2 (CASE)
ISBN 0-13-299736-3 (PAPER)

Parker Publishing Company
Career & Personal Development
West Nyack, New York 10995

Simon & Schuster, A Paramount Communications Company

Printed in the United States of America

Also by Mildred Carter

Helping Yourself with Foot Reflexology
Hand Reflexology: Key to Perfect Health

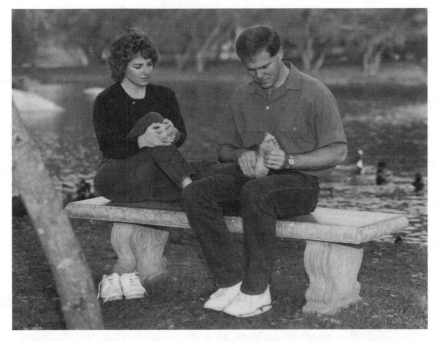

Photo "A": Reflexology is a simple, refreshing way to keep health in harmony with Nature. It requires NO expensive equipment or facilities.

Acknowledgments

Love and thanks to my family and friends, and the many chiropractors, naturopathic physicians, and medical doctors who have given their time and support in helping me complete this book.

I would especially like to thank my daughter, Tammy, for her invaluable help with the revision of this book. I also offer special thanks to my grandchildren—Brian, Sandy, Sherry, and Kevin—and to Gordon, Cindy, Christina, Chelsea, Malery, and Roy and Jennifer for their cheerfulness and help with photography.

Thanks to Stirling Enterprises, Inc., Cottage Grove, Oregon, for use of the reflex devices that were used as models.

With fondness, and thanks, I appreciate all of *you*, my students, fellow reflexologists, and readers. It is my privilege and pleasure to have the opportunity to share with you this natural way to perfect health. I hope reflexology will be your path to abundant mental energy and excellent physical health. May you and your loved ones live a life full of love and happiness.

Introduction

How You Can Feel Good All over Instantly

Reflexology is a sensational, dynamic, yet simple approach to glowing health. It requires no expense, no special equipment, no drugs, and no medication. Through reflex massage, you will be able to eliminate the causes and symptoms of sickness and pain from virtually every part of the body. Reflexology is simple and safe for anyone to use, anywhere, and at any time. The powerful healing forces of reflexology will make you whole; bring you renewed vigor, vitality, and beauty; and eliminate illness and pain from your life.

Your body is held together by the same energy forces that hold the stars, the moon, and the sun in their places. It is controlled by what is the equivalent of an electrical system with many "on" and "off" switches. There are "main circuits" to every organ, gland, and nerve, and these circuits have endings, or pressure points, in your hands, feet, and other parts of your body. By massaging, or working, these pressure points, you not only stop pain, but you also send a healing force to all parts of the body by opening up closed "electrical lines" that have shut off the universal life force. When these life lines are closed or clogged, malfunctioning glands and organs make you ill.

Reflexology gets to the cause of a problem by restoring the energy flow to the body's many different systems and functions. I will show you how to massage the reflexes on certain parts of your body to tap the healing current and to bring natural and prompt relief from practically all aches and pains, chronic or acute.

Through reflexology, I have discovered that there is a force within us that can heal; we can reach out with our hands and send healing radiation surging into the energy field of another person. Most of us, however, have not developed this power to its full capacity. In this book, I will show you how you can use your power through reflexology to heal yourself and others and realize almost instant results.

You will learn methods and techniques that will enable you to stop headaches, toothaches, and backaches within minutes, relieve constipation, sore throat, shortness of breath, heart pains, stomach problems, earaches, sciatica, hemorrhoids, childbirth pains, colds, flu, asthma, arthritis, and more. In this revised and expanded edition of the book, I have added chapters on premenstrual syndrome and menopause, cystic fibrosis and multiple sclerosis, losing weight naturally, eliminating mental and physical stress and tension, the importance of deep breathing, overcoming addictions, using reflexology with and for children, and reflexology and your pets.

Body reflexology also enables you to detect health problems before they become serious. You will gain more youthful energy and discover how to stay young well beyond your years. You will learn how to take a reflex break for a fast energy boost wherever you might be—in the office, shopping in a store, driving a car, or when the kids seem to be too much for you to handle.

Reflex massage starts the calming action that brings relief to tense nerves and knotted muscles. Within minutes, it banishes fatigue and sends a new vitality pulsing through your entire body. It seems to create a greater flow of blood throughout the body without undue strain, pressure, or overexertion of the heart. Thus, reflexology assists in the overall nourishment of the body.

I have spent many years travelling throughout the world, studying every method of natural healing that was available to me so that I might pass it on to you. I have learned many marvelous things about healing the body, making it beautiful, and renewing interest in life. But in all my studies of natural healing, I have never found one that compares to reflexology in bringing relief from most ailments. Yet reflexology is still unknown to too many people. That is why I wrote the original edition of *Body Reflexology*, and why I have updated and expanded it for the 1990s.

Other books on body reflex massage are complex and hard to understand. Here you will find the techniques of reflexology fully and simply illustrated by diagrams and photographs. In this new edition I have included more photographs and more detailed diagrams to make the techniques and methods of reflex massage even easier to use. In an effort to make reflexology as simple as possible for you, I have included only those reflexes that will benefit you the most.

No one should depend completely on reflexology as a cure-all. There are times when a medical doctor may be needed. However, reflexology is an effective alternative method for treating many illnesses and alleviating pain. A person is a structural, chemical, and spiritual being, and with reflex massage, you will learn how to bring all three elements into balance so that you can treat a whole person, rather than just a part of his or her body. If every part of the body is not in balance, there can be no complete relief from pain and illness.

Reflexology is truly magic, but you don't need a magician to make it work for you or anyone else. The power is right in your own hands. Use it today and every day to eliminate pain and illness from your life, and from the lives of those you love and all others you want to help.

A Word from the Author

Since the publication in 1983 of the first edition of *Body Reflexology*, I have received hundreds of letters from people all over the world who have discovered the great healing powers of reflex massage. Using the simple, special techniques of reflexology described in my book, these people have found cures for almost every type of ailment, and their lifestyles have changed dramatically. They have more vitality and stamina, are less depressed, and are more self-confident.

The body has an amazing capacity to heal itself. The keys to this renewed health are vigorous blood circulation, complete relaxation, daily activity, and proper diet. As this new edition of my book will show you, reflexology contributes to all these critical elements by helping the body resist illness and combat the discomforts of most health problems.

I have made audiotapes for the blind that describe in detail the reflexology techniques found in my books. I hope these tapes will be as helpful to those who cannot see as my books have been to those who can. The purpose of these tapes is not to restore sight, but to help the blind understand and use reflex massage to bring relief from pain and other health problems.

I fondly express my dedication and appreciation to those of you who wrote to me with such miraculous testimonials describing how reflexology has helped you or someone in your life. You may find your personal story here within this book. I do, however, respect your privacy and have, therefore, identified you by your initials only. The one exception to this is the correspondence from Bobby Chee, who so graciously gave his permission for me to use a few of his spectacular cases in Malaysia. [[Author: This credit to Bobby Chee is still applicable?]]

I thank you and am always delighted to hear from you.

Mildred Carter

Table of Contents

CHAPTER 1

How Reflexology Works to Help the Body Heal Itself

More than twenty million Americans have seen the effectiveness of reflexology on TV and have read of this natural technique of healing in many national magazines as well as in most newspapers. It is sometimes described under different names, but all these methods use the technique of pressing on certain points of the body.

I have proved beyond any doubt whatever the healing power of reflex massage in my books *Hand Reflexology: Key to Perfect Health* and *Helping Yourself with Foot Reflexology*.

Now we will take you a step further with the wonders of body massage which will also bring miracles of healing into your life and the lives of those you love.

Body reflexology will start the functioning of many processes throughout the whole body and leave nothing unattended when you follow the directions given.

You will release the healing power of the lymphatic system by opening up the flow of lymph fluid into damaged areas. You will speed up the healing forces by activating the nervous system when you massage the reflexes as directed and balance the vital energies among all the various systems.

Glance for a moment at Diagram 1. Notice how energy and circulation are slowed down when there is blockage in the line. We start health flowing back into our bodies by breaking up this blockage and letting the life energy flow freely to all parts of the body.

A tender spot any place on your body indicates a point of congestion in the energy lines, which in turn means trouble in some area that may be far removed from the tender point.

Now you can see why reflexology works such miracles of healing. This simple miracle of magic healing has been overlooked for many years because of its very simplicity.

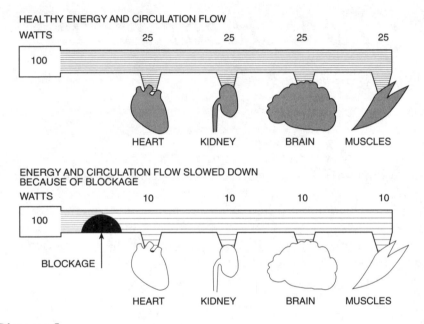

Diagram 1

A Medical Doctor Is Convinced

Mrs. Carter's explanation of why her reflexology works clashes so much with what I or any other physician who has studied the nervous system believe, that my first reaction to her book was anything but positive. But then I remembered the wisdom of a saying, "Why something works is not as important as whether it does work." The "why's" of any working method can be changed, but no "why" can help any *not working* method to perform.

So, I put Mrs. Carter to the test of trying reflexology on several people and found, to my surprise, that everything in her book was verified. Now I do not doubt the efficacy of this method.

—Dr. Van S.

How Reflexology Works

The press of a finger on a certain "button" (nerve ending) on the body may result in an odd tingling sensation in quite a different area, and you will know that the reflex button is connected with this remote part. Hold it for a few seconds; if it is sensitive, press it several times. You now have proof that the healing pressure on a reflex is getting through to the source of the trouble.

Sometimes the tingling will be felt where you least expect it. This doesn't always happen, but when it does you will be aware that you have discovered a life-giving current of health. It is this reward that makes reflex massage so valuable. It covers all parts of the body and brings them under control. It keeps corrosion from forming and causing trouble later on.

Don't be impatient. You must keep in mind that it has taken a long time for you to get into your present condition. Now you must give nature some time to correct it, although often the improvement is so rapid that it does seem like a miracle.

In some cases it is necessary to use prolonged stimulation to alleviate the pain, sometimes from twenty minutes to an hour. So don't give up if the pain does not subside immediately. It will work!

Treat the Slightest Twinge of Pain

Whenever you feel a pain anywhere in your body, even the slightest twinge of a pain, no matter where it is located, press and massage it *immediately*! It is the body's method of sending you a signal via the reflexes that there is trouble. Someplace there is a blockage causing malfunctioning to a certain area in the body. It may be far removed from the messenger sending the signal, but press the button now and you may prevent future illness from striking unexpectedly later on. Listen to your body. You will always get a warning signal before illness strikes, so heed it as you would a red light at a street crossing. *Stop* and press the reflex button, and you will continue to live free from illness.

Scientific Evidence
That Reflexology Works

Ever since acupuncture was introduced to the western world, interested doctors have sought to find scientific proof that stimulation of certain points in the body stops pain and helps heal illnesses. (By "scientific proof" we mean that which is obtained under controlled laboratory conditions.)

Recent research in France, Israel, Great Britain, Scotland, Canada, the United States, and other western countries has produced a number of discoveries that throw light on the way reflexology as well as acupuncture may work.

Dr. Roger Dalet, a specialist at Beaujon Hospital in Paris, tells us in his book, *How to Give Relief from Pain by the Simple Pressure of a Finger*, that stimulation of certain acupuncture points (which are the same as reflexology points) causes the blood to become enriched and leads to a marked improvement in respiratory function, particularly in asthmatic patients. Patients with disturbed heart rhythms show a marked improvement after acupuncture.

Dr. Dalet goes on to describe recordings of the movements of the stomach and intestines, called peristalsis. These have revealed that when peristalsis has been excessive—which may become very painful—the application of acupuncture needles in the front of the abdomen has brought about a considerable reduction of activity and a general calming of the system.

In this book I will show you how to accomplish the same results by using pressure on certain points instead of the acupuncture needles.

SCIENCE EXPLAINS WHY REFLEXOLOGY WORKS

The reflex points are energy junctions that relay and reinforce energy along meridian lines of the body, passing energy toward the organs and the nervous system.

Dr. Becker and his colleagues have been experimenting and testing with electrodes and have come up with scientific proof that electrical current passes most readily along the body's meridian lines. This proves that there are specific electrical properties at the reflex points and along the meridians that are different from the surrounding tissues.

After many months of testing at Aberdeen University and the University of California at La Jolla, a series of chemical messengers in the brain, chemically very similar to the drug morphine, were discovered. They are called endorphines and they have the same effect as morphine in suppressing pain. They seem to work by blocking the transmission of pain impulses from one neuron to another.

A number of these substances, all rather similar chemically, have now been discovered. They are known to have a calming or even euphoric effect, producing optimism and even joy, according to their chemical structure and the part of the brain affected.

A Canadian scientist, Professor Pomeranz of Toronto, made the discovery that acupuncture liberated these very endorphines. Reflexology accomplishes the same effect using pressure instead of needles.

MANY HAVE BEEN HELPED

Working the reflexes to help nature open channels of health to any and all parts of the body has proven very successful, and will not fail if properly applied. Reflexology not only helps nature open up these channels when congested, but also sends a supply of magnetic vital life force charging through the channels within the body like a healing shock wave.

In helping you to understand the simplicity of reflexology, I will ask you to recall a time in your life when you may have felt an electrical "signal" surging through your nerves. This may have been a time when you were suddenly frightened, or told by a dentist that you needed a tooth pulled; it may have been when just few of your hairs were pulled . . . whatever the instance, the signal in the nerves was very definite. The feeling most likely went through your entire body, from head to toe.

This is a good example of how electrical life energy travels through the nerve circuits when reflexology is used. However, with this dynamic healing power, one cannot usually "feel" the healing life force that provides such complete (and, in some cases, immediate) relief.

I have received hundreds of letters from people all over the world telling of sensational cures of nearly every type of illness using reflexology. Here are letters from a few who were helped.

Artificial Hip Pain Helped

Dear Ms. Carter:

I am a firm believer in the lack of using any pills. I was relieved of the reliance on drugs (prescribed by my family doctor) by acupuncture. I very seldom even use an aspirin. When I read your book on reflexology, you can imagine that I agreed with it 100%. I have used it on myself often.

My wife was a non-believer in reflexology. She has all kinds of problems. The other day she let me work on her feet. She felt immediate relief. Especially in the area where she has had an artificial hip inserted. She also has suffered from swelling. After working on her feet, the swelling has gone down so she can see her ankle shape after just one treatment. She still can't believe it, but she can't deny the proof that it works either.

I am a school teacher and this seems to me to be a very rewarding avenue. I like to be kept busy, and also like to help others. This might provide both, and be very rewarding.

Most Sincerely,

—Mr. S.F.R.

Eighty-Six Year Old Well and Happy

Dear Ms. Carter:

Thank you for writing your books. In my youth I was in the theater and had beautiful golden blond hair. For thirty years I colored my hair with an artificial product. Yet after using reflexology on my hands, feet and body, as well as buffing my fingernails . . . my hair has turned from grey to a more attractive color. Three years ago I was informed that I had cataracts, two years ago they were worse . . . but this year they are back to normal.

I could not walk well, I had been so bad that I brought an electric scooter. I used reflexology on myself and can now walk for 15 minutes without pain . . . anyone want a scooter?

When I was 76 years old I had to have a triple by-pass, but today I feel like I am 60. While I watch TV, I exercise my fingers aggressively on my head, feet, hands and body . . . the body tingles and this 86 year old is well and happy.

Sincerely,

—Mrs. G.B.

Reflexology Helps Seaman as He Sails Around the World

Dear Mrs. Carter,

May God give you more power to help people through your wonderful books, not only in the U.S.A., but throughout the whole world. I am a seaman, working on an international ship going around the world. And by chance, I came across your book "Hand Reflexology," somewhere in Korea.

Your book truly revealed the amazing health secret which triggers dynamic healing power of the body's mysterious *"nerve circuits"*. Recently, when I joined the ship in Malta, I encountered tremendous aches in my left and right ankles which nearly paralized me. If you can imagine, I was afraid I could not do the work in the ship; but because of your book, which I brought with me, I worked the reflexes mentioned. Little by little the pain moved out and I was able to walk normally, and now I am feeling well. I firmly believe that reactivating the reflexes is very effective!

I am so indebted to you Mrs. Carter, for sharing this method of physical healing and (maybe) the only way I can repay you is to tell and prove to others, including all my relatives and friends, what your book can do for us. Once more my sincere regards to you.

Very Respectfully Yours,

—A.M.M.

Reflexology Helped on Eighty-three-Year-Old

Dear Mrs. Carter,

I want to tell you about the wonderful results I am having with body massage. I am eighty-three years young, and thanks to you, my dear, I am young. Before you told me about the reflexes in the body I was hardly able to get around. I didn't have enough strength to get enough pressure on my feet and hands, although it did help some. I decided to try your complete method of working the reflexes in my body and, praise God, I could do it and feel the results. I just put all of my fingers together on both hands and pressed in deep where I needed relief, which was in most of my body. I could actually feel the healing working. How wonderful reflexology is and how wonderful I feel again. I think I will find a young husband!

I am sure you were placed on this earth to help God's people who are so in need of his natural methods of healing. Keep it up, my prayers are with you.

—Mrs. N.M.

Letter from a Minister

Dear Mrs. Carter,

I want to tell you what I have done with reflexology. After my sermon one Sunday I told my congregation that I was going to show those who were interested how to regain their health and keep it by using natural methods. I had everyone massage certain reflexes in their hands and then I had them take off their shoes and showed them certain reflexes in their feet. They love it. That was one month ago; I wish you could see the difference in my people now. Many of them are much healthier and in brighter spirits. Every day someone comes to tell me of the wonderful results they are having since I showed them the miracle of massaging the reflexes.

Reflexology is truly a miracle from God that we have had with us all the time.

We pray for you every day, we thank God and we thank you for the miracle of reflexology.

—Rev. D.W.

Techniques for Pressing Reflexes All Over the Body

In describing how to use reflexes found all over the body, it is best to start with those found in the hands and feet.

Place your thumb in the center of your palm or in the center of the bottom of your foot and, with a rotating motion, press and roll the thumb as if you were trying to break up lumpy sugar. Do this about five times; then move to another spot. You can tell which reflex you are massaging by studying Diagrams 2, 3, 4, and 5. You are *not* to rub the *skin* but the reflexes *under the skin*. Use this method for massaging reflexes, except where instructed to hold a steady pressure.

A more advanced method of massaging the hands and the feet involves starting to rub the thumb or the big toe, then completely massaging every finger and every toe, searching for tender reflexes. Don't just use your fingers here. Use a device like a pencil or the little hand reflex probe described in the chapter on reflex devices. Roll this between every toe on both sides and also between every finger. You will be amazed at the "ouch" spots you will discover in these areas.

In Diagrams 6A, 6D, and 6E, you will find that there are also important reflexes on the tops of the feet and on the backs of the hands. Be sure to massage these reflex buttons to stimulate many areas in the body. Hold a steady, firm pressure for a slow count of seven, and then release for a count of three. Do this three times more on the calves of the legs for about 15 minutes to alleviate pain throughout the entire body. See Diagram 6H.

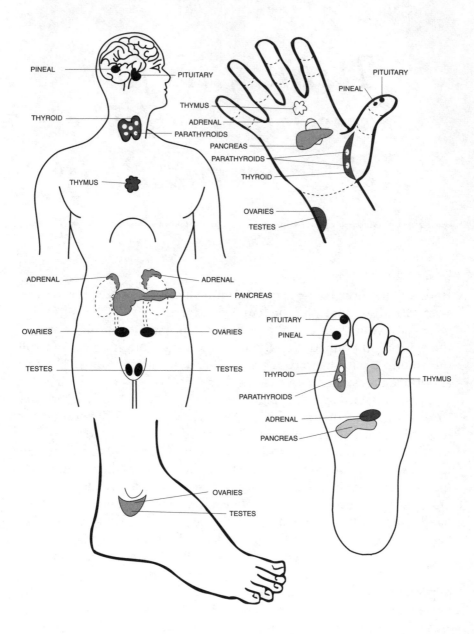

Diagram 2

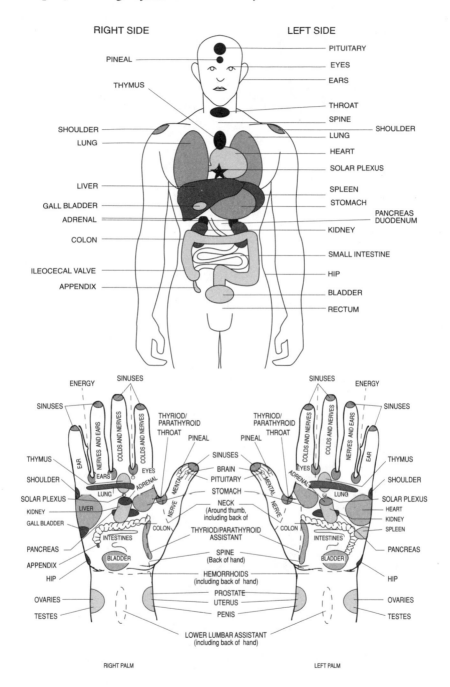

RIGHT SIDE   LEFT SIDE

PITUITARY
PINEAL
EYES
EARS
THYMUS
THROAT
SPINE
SHOULDER
SHOULDER
LUNG
LUNG
HEART
SOLAR PLEXUS
LIVER
SPLEEN
GALL BLADDER
STOMACH
ADRENAL
PANCREAS
DUODENUM
COLON
KIDNEY
SMALL INTESTINE
ILEOCECAL VALVE
HIP
APPENDIX
BLADDER
RECTUM

ENERGY   SINUSES   SINUSES   ENERGY
SINUSES   SINUSES
NERVES AND EARS
COLDS AND NERVES
COLDS AND NERVES
THYRIOD/
PARATHYROID
THROAT
THYRIOD/
PARATHYROID
THROAT
PINEAL   PINEAL
COLDS AND NERVES
COLDS AND NERVES
NERVES AND EARS
THYMUS
SINUSES
THYMUS
EAR
BRAIN
EAR
SHOULDER
PITUITARY
SHOULDER
EARS   EYES
ADRENAL
STOMACH
EYES   ADRENAL
SOLAR PLEXUS
LUNG
NERVE   MENTAL
MENTAL   NERVE
LUNG
SOLAR PLEXUS
KIDNEY
NECK
HEART
LIVER
(Around thumb,
KIDNEY
GALL BLADDER
including back of
SPLEEN
COLON
THYRIOD/PARATHYROID
COLON
PANCREAS
ASSISTANT
PANCREAS
INTESTINES
INTESTINES
APPENDIX
SPINE
BLADDER
(Back of hand)
BLADDER
HIP
HEMORRHOIDS
HIP
(including back of hand)
OVARIES
PROSTATE
OVARIES
UTERUS
TESTES
PENIS
TESTES

LOWER LUMBAR ASSISTANT
(including back of hand)

RIGHT PALM   LEFT PALM

Diagram 3

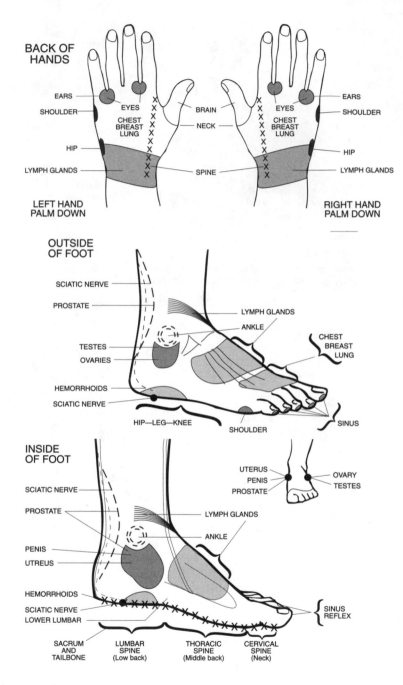

Diagram 4

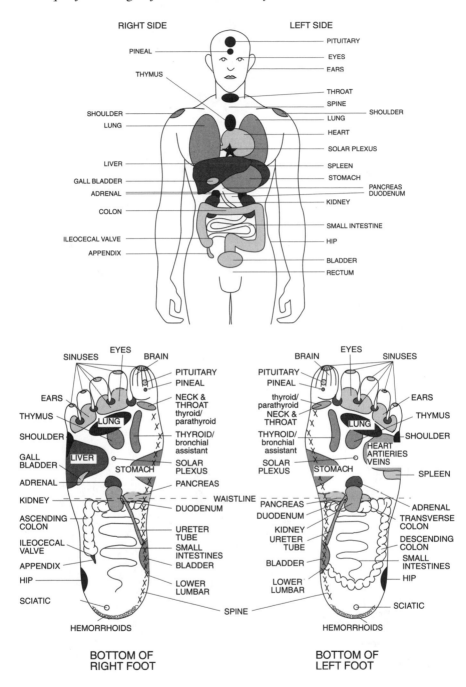

Diagram 5

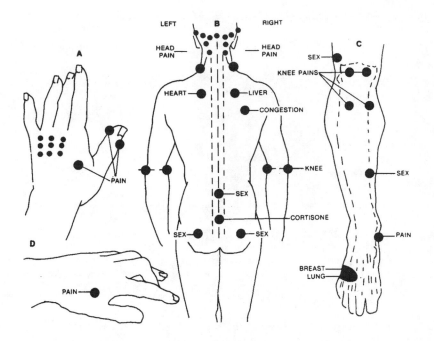

This diagram shows several pain control reflex buttons that are stimulated by pressure that causes them to release natural pain-inhibiting chemicals in the brain called "endorphines." Also shown are energy-stimulating reflex buttons in various locations.

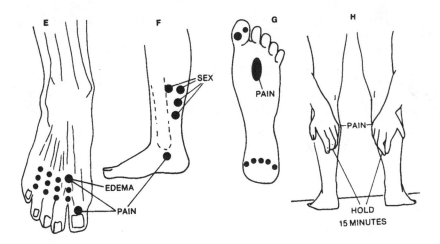

Diagram 6

The Electrical Power in Your Hands

The palm of the right hand is positive and stimulates energy, which has a strengthening effect.

The palm of the left hand is negative and has a sedating, soothing, and cleaning effect.

The use of both hands will give you the combined effect of both energies.

The backs of the hands have the opposite electrical energy from the palms. The back of the right hand will be negative and the back of the left hand will be positive.

The back of the head is positive while the front of the head is negative. If you place the palm of your right hand on the lower part of the back of your head and place the palm of the left hand on the front part of the head, you will be enforcing the natural energies of the head, and a feeling of well-being and strength will be the result. If you reverse this procedure, you will have a lowering of the efficiency of the brain, which will have a disturbing effect.

So remember, when you are pressing a reflex button to stop pain, try to use the left hand. If you are using a reflex implement for pain, hold it in your left hand. If you are seeking to send the energized healing forces to slow, stagnated, and clogged areas in the body, you may gain better results by using the strengthening effect of the right hand.

Reflexology is a natural method of healing, no matter where or how it is used, but it is more effective if you are aware of the positive and negative electrical power in your hands.

A Husband's Life Is Prolonged

Dear Mrs. Carter,

The doctors said my husband had less than one week to live. After talking to you I started to give him reflexology on his whole body. I had your books on foot and hand reflexology, which helped keep him alive. Then I advanced to body reflexology and he lived for four more years. The doctors think I am crazy to use reflexology, but it did for him what they could not do, and I am still alive and healthy today thanks to reflexology.

—M.L.

BODY REFLEXES

You can see by studying the diagrams that follow that, unlike the reflexes in the hands and the feet, body reflexes do not always follow a straight meridian line. There are *several* reflex points located in certain areas of the body that will stimulate renewed life to more than one malfunctioning area.

So, we will have to use a somewhat new technique when using the body reflexes. Because these reflex buttons are sometimes in hard-to-massage areas, it is difficult to give simple directions.

By studying the diagrams, you will see what I mean. In Diagram 12, notice how many reflexes are located in just a portion of the head. How are you going to find a specific button? Hence some new techniques come into play. You will find photos of most of them. Sometimes it may be necessary to ask another person for help.

Look at Diagrams 7 and 8. You will see reflex points scattered over various parts of the body. Now turn to Diagrams 9, 10, and 11. Many of you are not familiar with the glands and organs within the body; I would like you to study the positions of these glands and organs so you will be able to associate them with certain reflex buttons when you are instructed to massage them for specific ailments.

HOW TO WORK BODY REFLEXES FOR THE MOST EFFECTIVE RESULTS

Look at Diagrams 3 and 5. Note how the reflex buttons are located more or less over the glands and organs they represent. To press these specific reflex points, use the middle finger, which has the strongest energy flow, or use the four-finger method, which sometimes seems to have the power of a laser beam. There are several ways in which you can massage (or work) these sensitive reflex buttons. All reflex buttons not named on the charts are energy stimulants and important to many areas of the body. You will find many tender reflex buttons that are not marked. Don't let this worry you. If they are sending an "ouch" signal, this means that some place in your body is in trouble and is asking for your help. So work it out.

It is best to start by massaging the *important* reflexes located in various places over the entire body.

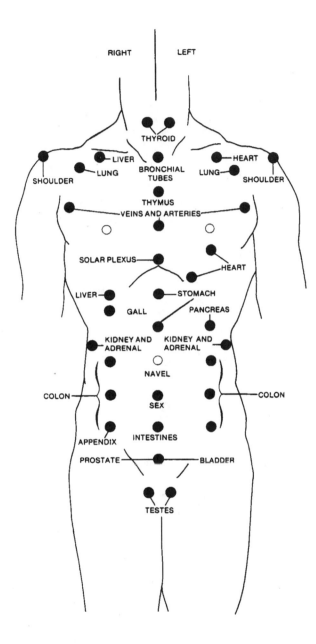

Diagram 7

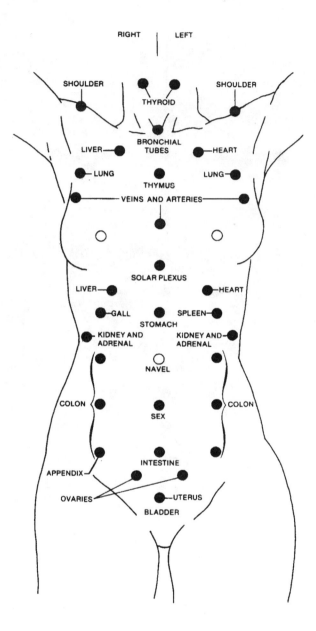

Diagram 8

MIRROR IMAGE

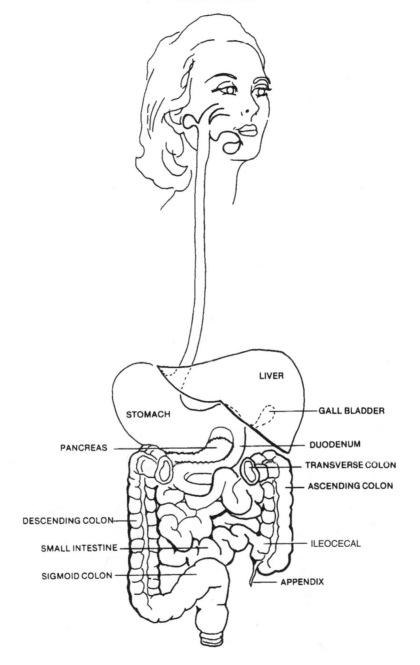

LIVER

GALL BLADDER

STOMACH

DUODENUM

PANCREAS

TRANSVERSE COLON

ASCENDING COLON

DESCENDING COLON

SMALL INTESTINE

ILEOCECAL

SIGMOID COLON

APPENDIX

Diagram 9

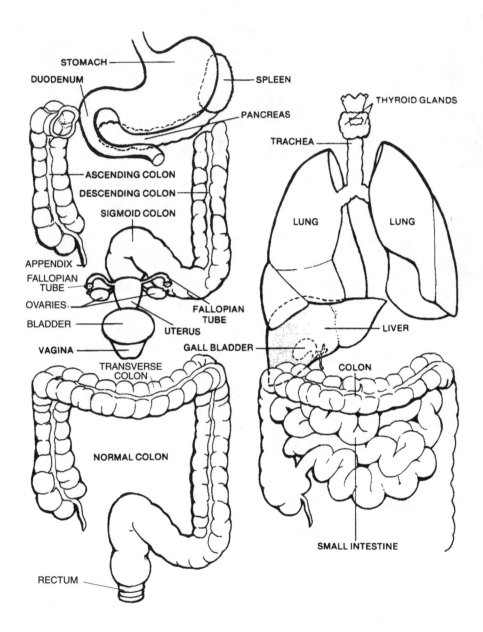

STOMACH
DUODENUM
SPLEEN
THYROID GLANDS
PANCREAS
TRACHEA
ASCENDING COLON
DESCENDING COLON
SIGMOID COLON
LUNG
LUNG
APPENDIX
FALLOPIAN TUBE
OVARIES
FALLOPIAN TUBE
BLADDER
UTERUS
VAGINA
LIVER
GALL BLADDER
TRANSVERSE COLON
COLON
NORMAL COLON
SMALL INTESTINE
RECTUM

Diagram 10

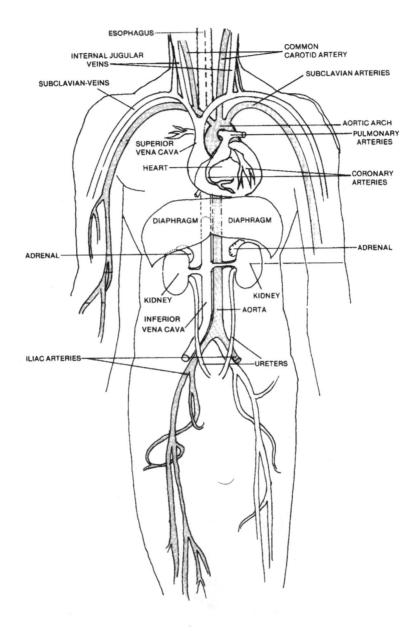

ESOPHAGUS

COMMON CAROTID ARTERY

INTERNAL JUGULAR VEINS

SUBCLAVIAN ARTERIES

SUBCLAVIAN-VEINS

AORTIC ARCH

PULMONARY ARTERIES

SUPERIOR VENA CAVA

HEART

CORONARY ARTERIES

DIAPHRAGM   DIAPHRAGM

ADRENAL

ADRENAL

KIDNEY   KIDNEY

AORTA

INFERIOR VENA CAVA

ILIAC ARTERIES

URETERS

Diagram 11

Use the middle finger to press lightly on each reflex button. If it is painful, you will know that there is congestion somewhere. Let us say that you find a painful button over the stomach area. This does not necessarily mean that the stomach is the organ in trouble. When you look at Diagrams 7 and 8, you can see that tender reflexes could be sending out pain signals from other malfunctioning nerves or tissue in a congested area. If it hurts when pressed, assume that there is a blocked line that is slowing down the electrical life force to a congested area. Hold pressure on this reflex button until the hurt subsides or for seven seconds at a time. Keep in mind that you are doing more than diagnosing areas of malfunction when you massage these reflexes that are giving you warning signals of congestion or malfunctioning of a certain organ, gland, or tissue. You are also treating the *ailment*, restoring health by releasing the blockage to the energy field.

On the chest and abdomen, we will use finger pressure to massage the reflexes. See Photos 1, 2, 3, 4, and 5. However, some people like to use a device called the reflex roller in these areas. See Photos 6 and 7. I will explain how to use the reflex implements in a later chapter.

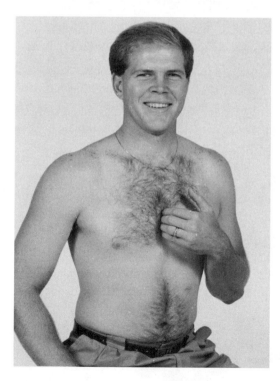

Photo 1: Position for pressing reflexes to the thymus, veins, and arteries.

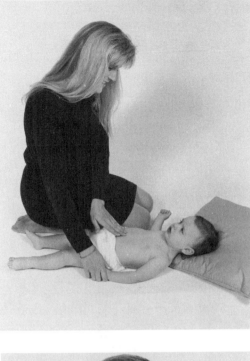

Photo 2: A light pressure on the stomach of a child to help an upset stomach, etc.

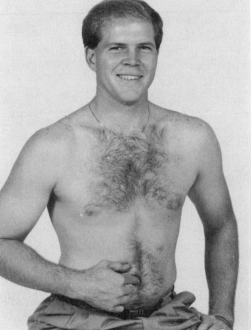

Photo 3: Pressing finger into the navel to energize the whole body.

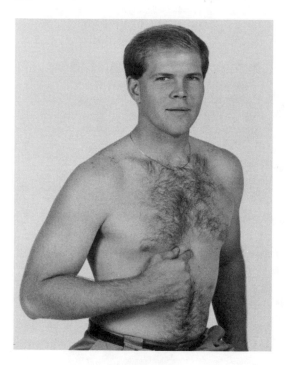

Photo 4: Pressing finger on reflexes to stomach to relieve painful ulcers and other stomach problems.

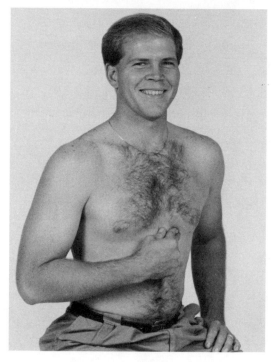

Photo 5: Pressing one of the reflex buttons for the heart.

Body Reflexology Aids a Woman Who Lives Alone

Dear Mrs. Carter,

I want to thank you for telling me about reflexology. I am seventy-three years old and live by myself out in the country. I have always been very healthy so I don't mind living so far from people. Then I got to feeling bad, and it seemed that all at once my body didn't function well. I felt worse and worse every day, so I decided to call you. I had used reflexology for many years to stay healthy. Now I needed to know what was wrong.

After you explained about body reflexology and told me how to use it along with the foot and hand massages, I have completely recovered and feel better than ever. My friends did talk me into going to a doctor after you told me I should. He said I was in perfect health, younger than my years, and he told me that whatever I was doing, to keep doing it.

I am so grateful to you. Thank you again, dear lady.

—M.G.

Using the Reflex Pulse Test on the Abdomen

With the middle finger, or using all fingers held together on one or both hands, press into your navel firmly but gently. To get the full benefit from this test, you should lie on your back. If you have a pad of fat over the abdominal area, then you will have to use the fingers to press in deeply through the fat pad. Now, feel for a pulse beat. Do you feel the pulse throb? If you do, this indicates that there is trouble in this area and it needs help. How do you give it help? Hold pressure on this reflex for the count of seven. Then use a slight rotary movement, keeping the fingers on the area of the pulse beat.

Now we will go to other reflex buttons in the abdomen. Look at Diagrams 7 and 8. Using this same test method with the finger, feel each indicated reflex button for the beat of the pulse. If you cannot find a pulse beat, you can be happy to know that this area is free from trouble. If you do feel the throb of the pulse, then you know that it means malfunctioning of the organ or trouble in the zone for this reflex point.

Remember to sedate all reflexes that are painful on light pressure by holding to the count of seven. If you have to press in deeply to feel the throb of the pulse, you should stimulate the point by using heavier pressure. Many of these reflexes may be quite painful when pressed. By pressing and massaging these "ouch" points, you will be amazed at how quickly the pain subsides. Usually this happens while you are using the reflex pressure system. It will really amaze you when you feel the pain disappear under your very fingertips. You will have performed a miracle of healing, for, when the pulse can no longer be felt and the pain under your fingers has subsided, it means that the problem in the corresponding organ also has subsided. You have released the healing forces of nature to revive glandular activity!

Morning Reflexology Test

Before you get up each morning take a reflexology test by pressing reflex buttons in the abdomen and the chest. This will not only be a test for danger signals but it will stimulate your organs and glands and help prevent any congestion that might be accumulating along life lines to parts all over the body.

When the pain stops at the point of finger pressure, you will know that tension has been released and you will also feel that the pain coming from another part of the body has subsided. When you arise, you will have a feeling of energy and well-being that you have not felt for a long time.

I want you to do these exercises every morning, not only to *put* you in good health but also to *keep* you feeling full of energy and in perfect health for the rest of your long life.

If you can feel the pulse or a hurt in a certain reflex spot, use a rotary motion with the finger for a few seconds to help dissipate the painful reflex button.

Now, we will assume that you are lying down on your back with your abdomen exposed. Place your middle finger in your navel and feel for a pulse beat. See Photo 2. After holding this position for the count of seven, massage around the navel using all the fingers except the thumb. Now with the palm of the hand, start massaging at the navel in a clockwise motion, and work outward in an ever-larger circle until you are massaging the whole abdomen. Do this three times; then repeat counterclockwise. You can see how the energy of your hand will stimulate the entire abdominal area. Remember, when pain radiates from the navel to other parts of the body, the massage is not only a test but also a treatment for ailing parts of the body.

The Ice Cube Technique

When working any of the reflex buttons that seem to resist full recovery, you might try using the ice cube method. Use the same rotary motion on the tender reflex button with the corner of an ice cube. Press it on the sore button for about three seconds, then lay the hand on the spot for a second, then repeat with the ice cube once more.

Reflexes on the Chest

Now, proceed to the reflex points on the chest. See Photos 1, 5, and 6. Use the same massage technique on these reflex buttons as you did on the abdomen, except you will find that these reflex buttons will be located mostly over bone and muscle so that you will not press the fingers in as deeply as you did on the abdomen. You will still hold a steady pressure to test for tender spots, using the rotating massage when you find an "ouch" button. In many cases, tapping several times with the fingers will give better results. Although many points pictured on the charts are special reflex buttons for specific glands and organs, feel for added reflex points as you cover the chest and abdomen with your fingertips. Many people like to use the reflex roller to help them locate tender reflexes that they might have overlooked when using only the fingers. See Photos 6 and 7.

A Boost of Electrical Energy

Now, before you get out of bed, buff your nails to give yourself a boost of electrical energy that will fill your whole being with an electrical radiance and will last you all day. See Photo 8. In my book, *Hand Reflexology: Key to Perfect Health*, I told how to buff the nails to stimulate the growth of new hair. Since then, I have had many reports of how it also stimulates renewed electrical energy and vitality to the whole body.

You will find a full explanation of how to buff the nails in the chapter on hair.

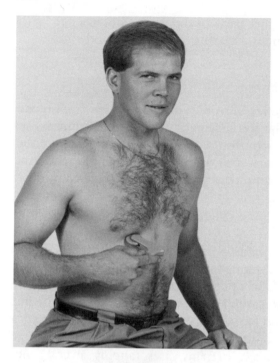

Photo 6: How to use reflex
roller to massage reflexes in
the chest area.

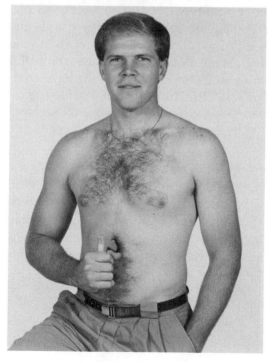

Photo 7: Using the reflex
roller massager to stimulate
abdominal reflexes.

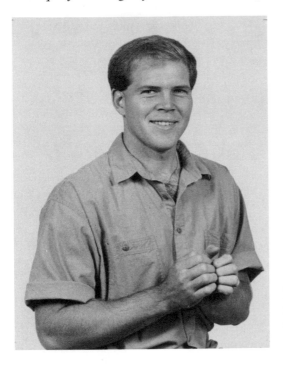

Photo 8: Position for buffing the nails to energize the whole body and promote the growth of hair.

CHAPTER 3

How to Use Special Exercises to Stimulate the Reflexes on the Head

Several diagrams of the head are included in this chapter. As you study them, you will be amazed at the many reflexes you will find and how they are related to all parts of your body.

When I give you specific directions on how to stimulate the reflexes, you will better understand their importance. You need not learn where all these reflexes are located by sight, but with a little practice you will learn their approximate locations by feel. This will hold true in most cases throughout this book. Study the diagrams and photos as we progress.

TECHNIQUE FOR MASSAGING THE REFLEXES ON THE HEAD

Study Diagrams 12, 13, and 14. Take note of how many important reflexes are located here. You do not need to remember where they are located; I will point these out to you as we need them further on in the book. I just want you to familiarize yourself with the importance of the different techniques of working the reflexes in the head.

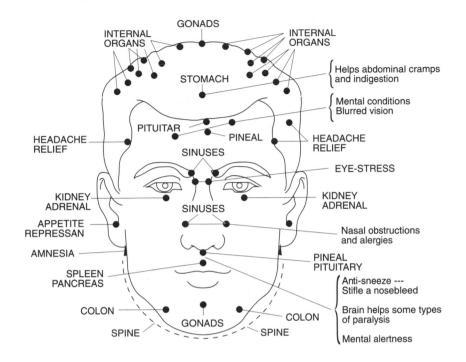

GONADS
INTERNAL ORGANS
INTERNAL ORGANS
STOMACH
Helps abdominal cramps and indigestion
Mental conditions Blurred vision
PITUITAR
PINEAL
HEADACHE RELIEF
SINUSES
HEADACHE RELIEF
EYE-STRESS
KIDNEY ADRENAL
SINUSES
KIDNEY ADRENAL
APPETITE REPRESSAN
Nasal obstructions and alergies
AMNESIA
SPLEEN PANCREAS
PINEAL PITUITARY
Anti-sneeze --- Stifle a nosebleed
COLON
GONADS
COLON
Brain helps some types of paralysis
SPINE
SPINE
Mental alertness

Diagram 12

Use your fingers to find special areas on the head. In Diagram 12, notice on the very center of the top of the head we find the reflexes to the reproductive organs. Down toward the forehead is the reflex to the stomach. Under the nose we find the reflex to the pineal and pituitary, then the spleen, and then the pancreas reflexes. Straight down from these reflexes we find the gonad reflexes on the chin. This seems to be on the center meridian line that runs through the body.

One way to massage these reflexes is to use the center finger, which is called the fire finger because it sends out energy more strongly than the other fingers. Press it on the center of the forehead just below the hair line. With a pressing, rolling motion feel for a sensitive spot. Do not rub the skin; rather, rub the bone area under the skin very gently. Now, move the finger down to the center of the forehead

Back of the Head

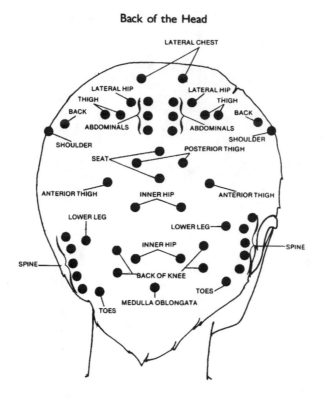

LATERAL CHEST

LATERAL HIP

THIGH

BACK

ABDOMINALS

SHOULDER

SEAT

ANTERIOR THIGH

INNER HIP

LATERAL HIP

THIGH

BACK

ABDOMINALS

SHOULDER

POSTERIOR THIGH

ANTERIOR THIGH

LOWER LEG

LOWER LEG

INNER HIP

SPINE

SPINE

INNER HIP

BACK OF KNEE

TOES

TOES

MEDULLA OBLONGATA

TOES

Diagram 13

and feel for another tender button, which will be a reflex to the pineal (commonly known as the third eye). Halfway between this spot and the bridge of the nose is another sensitive reflex that needs massage. This reflex affects the sinuses.

Massaging Only Certain Reflexes

This is one way to massage specific reflex buttons on the head. But you do not need to massage each and every one of these reflexes unless told to do so for a specific purpose later in the book. Other and easier methods of stimulating all these head and face reflexes more fully will be described later. But, for now, do note that head massages are very important.

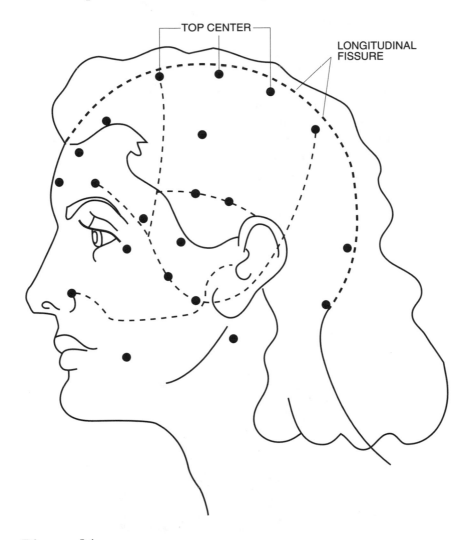

Diagram 14

Look at Diagram 13, illustrating the back of the head. Notice all the reflexes located here. Now go to Diagram 14 to see the location of the reflexes on the side of the head. You may have to refer back to these charts now and then when following directions for treating malfunctioning areas elsewhere in the body. We will use three different methods of stimulation.

Methods of Stimulation

1. Grab handfuls of hair and pull. This stimulates not only the hair but also the reflexes to the whole body. See Photo 9.

2. Close your fists very loosely and swing them loosely from the wrists as if they were on hinges. Very gently use these loose fists to tap the head. See Photo 10. Tap it all over very quickly. Do not do this for more than thirty seconds. This will be enough to bring life to every organ and gland in your body.

3. If you have a wire brush, use this to tap the head gently all over. See Photo 11. This is an excellent reflex stimulator and also stimulates the hair follicles to help promote a new and luxurious head of hair.

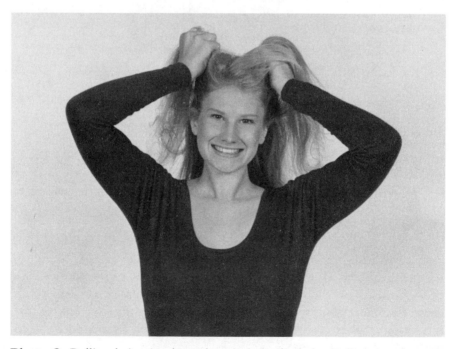

Photo 9: Pulling hair stimulates the whole body, helps indigestion, hangovers, etc.

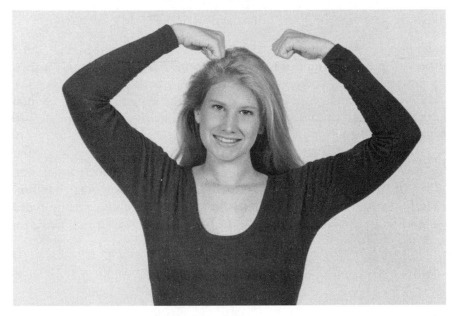

Photo 10: Lightly tap head to promote bladder function and good sexual activity, as well as other benefits.

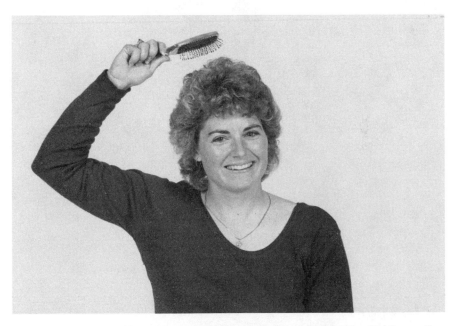

Photo 11: Tapping the head and body with the wire brush stimulates all the body reflexes.

ADJUSTMENT OF THE SKULL

The flow of cerebrospinal fluid is believed to be affected by the almost microscopic movement of the cranial bones during breathing. If these bones in the skull become stuck together, it is thought that the fluid will not be pumped well enough through the spinal column; the muscles will weaken because the energy related to the cerebrospinal fluid cannot flow freely.

Adjustment of the cranial bones should be left to a doctor who is familiar with this technique. But if you find that the abdominal muscles are weak, this may be due to the parietal bones being jammed together at the top of the head. To strengthen the abdominal muscles, you should massage the forehead as if to pull the skull apart along the seam. See Photo 12.

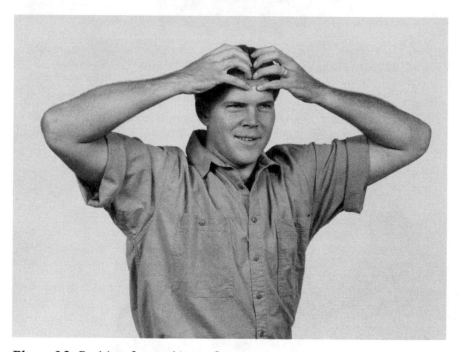

Photo 12: Position for working reflexes on head and forehead.

A car door once slammed on my head (my head had been caught between the top of the car and the door). I felt funny and had odd headaches for several days. I felt that the cranial bones had been jammed together. No doctors in the area were familiar with adjusting the skull, so I started to press and pull the cranial bones myself. After a few days I felt better and the uncomfortable sensations in my head stopped. This was several years ago, and I still feel fine.

THE ALL-IMPORTANT MEDULLA OBLONGATA

The medulla oblongata is a reflex button that we will use throughout this book. It is one of the magic buttons that will start your power generator into action. It will enable you to open up the electrical channels to all parts of the body. It will bring you release from daily nervous tensions when you need it. This button will generate almost instant energy. You decide on the action you want, and in seconds it is yours to command. This magic reflex button can be used at any time and in almost any location without anyone knowing what you are doing.

In Diagram 13 notice the button located in the hollow at the base of the skull on the back of the head. This is the medulla oblongata, a vitality-generating reflex button. It is the enlarged portion of the spinal cord, just after it enters the cranium. It is a giant controlling agent containing the cardiovascular center and the respirator center. It controls blood pressure and the dilation and constriction of blood vessels. It controls postural balance and the reflexes concerned with swallowing, vomiting, and many other actions. Even though the spinal cord is located on the inside of the skull, you will cause reactions whenever you apply any type of reflex therapy to it. The entire body network funnels impulses into the spinal cord. These messages are relayed to the power-manufacturing centers of the brain and body. The messages are sent to all the endocrine glands. See Chapter 8 and learn the importance of each one of these glands, how each gland is a producer of important hormones, and how each one of these glands is a source of health, beauty, vigor, and vitality.

The medulla oblongata reflex will give you instant go-power when it is needed. It is a very important reflex button and will be referred to many times in this book, so it is important that you learn the best technique for massaging it.

Technique of Reflex Massage

To turn on this sensational dynamo of action, find a little hollow between two muscle attachments at the base of the skull. See medulla oblongata, Diagram 13. Use either the middle finger of one hand or the middle fingers of both hands. You will have to use the method that is easiest for you. Now, put the finger or fingers into the hollow area and press. Is it painful? Feel it! Press it! Massage it! This is the fantastic magic reflex button that can give you the unlimited energy and go-power that everyone needs in these busy, stress-filled days.

SPECIAL BODY WARMER REFLEXES

As you study Diagram 14, you will see special points marked in various places on the side of the head. These are known as neurovascular receptors. I call them the body warmer reflexes to keep them simple and easy to remember. Each of these special reflexes is in a relative position. Remember that all heads are not the same shape, so you have to learn the approximate areas by searching for tender or sensitive points. With practice, you will learn to find them on yourself and others quite easily by reaching and feeling with your fingers. See Photos 12, 13, 14, 15, and 16 for different positions used to massage these body warmer reflexes on the head. These body warmer reflexes keep the lines open to special heaters in various parts of the body.

Let us liken the body warmers to little electric heaters that control the temperature of the entire body. If you are unable to adjust to temperature changes in the weather, some of your body heaters are not functioning properly and need to be reactivated.

These body warmers gather and regulate the energy of the digestive, sexual, and respiratory organs, and others. They work in cooperation with the lungs, the small intestines, the kidneys, the heart, and the sex organs.

The meridian of the body warmers begins at the root of the nail of the little finger and ascends up the back part of the body. If you will look once more at Diagram 14, you will better understand how the exercises that I give you to massage the head will help stimulate most, if not all, of the body warmer reflexes in the whole body.

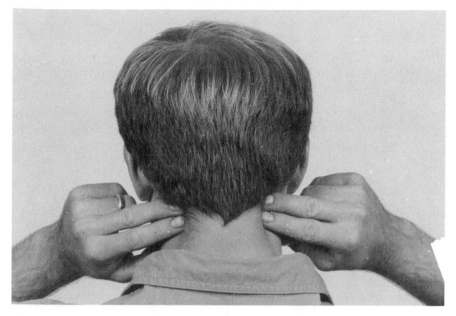

Photo 13: Pressing reflexes on the edge of the skull for headache and other complaints.

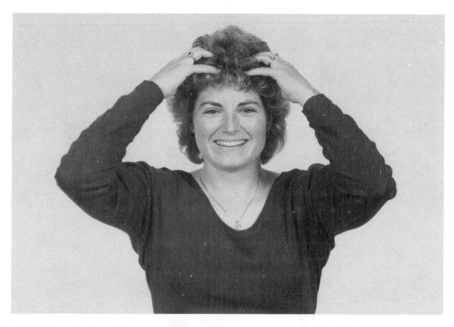

Photo 14: Position for pressing reflexes on top of head to energize areas in the whole body. Also benefits mental conditions.

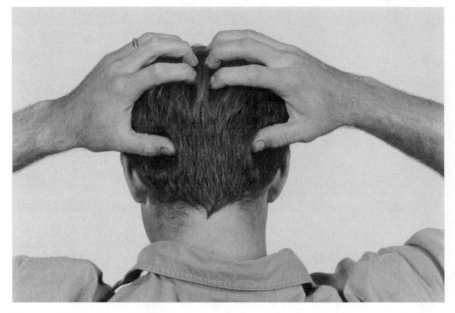

Photo 15: Position for massaging reflexes on back of head to energize many areas of the body.

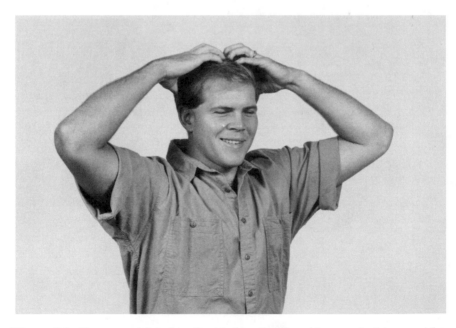

Photo 16: Shows position for stimulating the thyroid, gonads, lungs, and heart.

As we work the reflexes in other places of the body, we automatically press on and massage many of the body warmers without having to learn their exact locations. Keep in mind that if you find a tender reflex, no matter what part of the body it is getting a distress signal from, you should press and hold it until the hurt subsides.

CHAPTER 4

How to Use Reflexology on the Ears

As you can see in Diagram 15, there are many important reflexes in the ears. They will stimulate a renewed flow of life force into every part of your body when pressed, pulled, and massaged. The ears, like the hands and the feet, have reflexes for the entire body. Because of the relationship of the reflexes in the ears to the rest of the body, reflex massage of the ears can help to correct many symptoms of malfunctioning organs.

THE EAR AND ITS ACUPOINTS

The ear is a complex sense organ endowed with a hundred acupoints. Its accessibility makes it ideal for the acupuncturist, who uses needles for stimulation to promote health in the rest of the body.

We have now learned to use the fingers to stimulate these sensitive reflexes. People twist, pull, and pinch their ears unconsciously, especially the earlobes, when something perplexing bothers them. Thus, instinctively, people reinvent this wonderful healing technique.

Because there are some one hundred reflexes in the ears, it is almost impossible to pinpoint all of them, so let us do a few exercises to stimulate as many of them as possible.

THE EAR

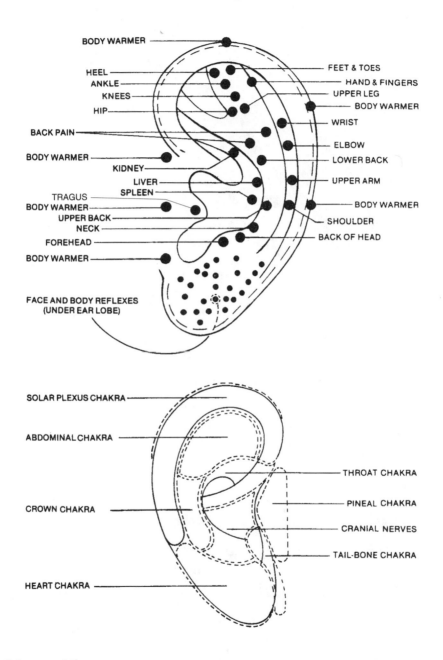

Diagram 15

See Photo 17. Place the fingers behind the ears and flatten them forward against the side of the head. Holding the ear with the third, fourth, and fifth fingers, tap the index finger on the ear to get a drum sound. Do this about five times to stimulate the gallbladder.

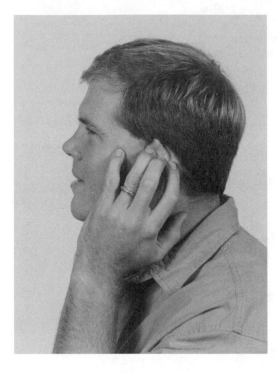

Photo 17: Bending the ear forward for tapping.

Now, place the cupped hand over one ear and tap gently with the other hand to get the sound of a seashell. This stimulates the kidneys and the triple-warmer organs.

Diagnosing Illness by Examining the Ears

Medical researchers tell us that the ear can be used to diagnose pain and illness in the rest of the body by observing temperature change and tenderness. Accuracy in ear diagnosis is said to be so good that an expert can achieve up to 90 percent accuracy in diagnosis of many conditions.

There are various changes in certain parts of the ear when specific areas of the body are stimulated. The ear can become very painful to the touch in a localized area corresponding to a specific part of the body.

Reflex pressure used on specific areas of the ear has been demonstrated on the stage, where almost immediate results were accomplished. The subjects who were worked on recovered from various illnesses almost immediately.

You may be able to find relief for malfunctioning areas in other parts of the body by using reflex pressure on specific buttons on the ear. See Diagram 15. Since the ear is such a small area to contain so many reflexes, you will have to use the press-and-feel technique. You might press with the fingernails or use reflex clamps. See Photos 18, 19, and 20.

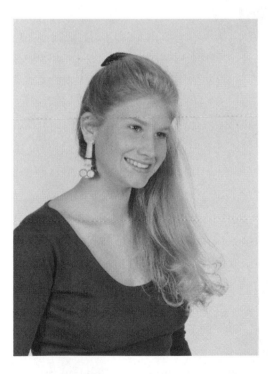

Photo 18: Reflex clamp on the right ear to anesthetize areas on the right side of the body.

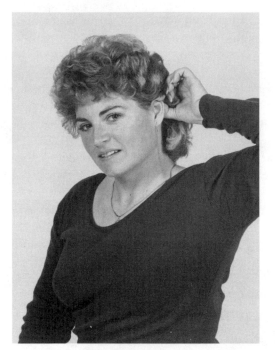

Photo 19: Massaging the reflexes in the ear for health and beauty.

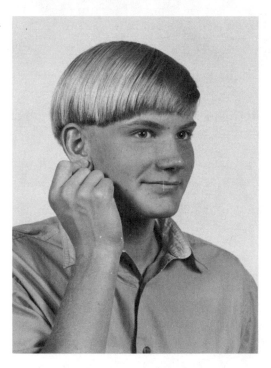

Photo 20: Children can learn to massage the reflexes in ears and other parts of the body to greatly benefit health.

Follow our motto, "If it is sore, rub it out," even if you don't know exactly what part of the body it corresponds to. If a certain point in the ear is painful to the touch, it means there is a health problem in some other area of the body that is sending a call for help. Somewhere a line is not getting its full supply of energy. By pressing the tender reflex in the ear, you are contacting another main circuit that will open up the line to full power. Remember to check the ear reflexes along with all other reflex points when you have health problems to overcome.

STIMULATING REFLEXES ON THE EARS

Reflex points on the ear slightly resemble the shape of the human fetus. The lobe of the ear represents the head—moving up the ear you will notice reflexes to body parts and on top of the lobe are reflexes to the feet.

Starting at the tops of the ears, pinch them between the thumbs and forefingers. Doing both ears at the same time, pinch this whole area using a pinch-and-roll technique. See Photo 19. You will probably find many tender reflexes as you progress along the entire ear. Tug the ears upward, keeping them close to the head. Lower your fingers to the narrow part of the ears, still using the pinch-and-roll method, and pull the ears out away from the head. Do this several times. Notice how they begin to tingle and burn.

Let us progress down to the lower lobes of the ears. Use the pinch-and-roll method of massage to pull, tug, and pinch these lobes for a few seconds. See Photo 20. Then, with the fingers, start at the top of the ear and pinch and roll the outer ridge all the way around to the lobes. Now hook the little fingers in the holes of the ears and pull out in all directions. End this massage by pinching and massaging the small flap (the tragus) located in front of the ear opening.

Now press the reflex buttons just behind the lobes of the ears, first on the bony section, then in the hollow. These also are magic reflex buttons that can free you from tension and cure sinus problems and headaches.

HOW TO HELP TINNITUS

Tinnitus is an upsetting problem caused by strange noises in the ears or the head. In some cases, it has been thought impossible to cure, but I believe that any kind of distress can be cured by nature. First, make sure there is no buildup of wax in the ear. See Diagram 15 and massage all the ear reflexes, giving special attention to reflexes labeled as body warmers and the reflex located under the earlobe. There are three body warmer reflexes for each ear in addition to the reflex on the hollow under the earlobes. Do both ears by pinching, rolling, and squeezing each reflex for the slow count of seven. See Photos 19 and 20.   •

Scuba Diver's Ears Helped by Reflexology

While waiting for a chartered boat in Hawaii, I started talking with a young girl sitting next to me in a coffee shop.

She told me that she taught deep sea and scuba diving, though she seemed young for that kind of work. She told me that her ears had become "scratched." That is the term divers use when the ear has been damaged from diving too deep or coming to the surface too quickly.

The inside of her head itched, so it nearly drove her mad sometimes, and she was told nothing could be done for it. I am always interested in learning what reflexology will do in unusual cases like this, so I asked her to let me have her hand for a moment. Because only the right ear was affected, I took her right hand and found the ring finger and the little finger to be tender. I massaged them a few seconds; you wouldn't believe the strange look that came into her eyes. She said, "It's stopped itching! I can't believe it. My head feels clear and normal. What did you do?"

I showed her where and how to massage the reflexes to the ears and told her to teach it to her diving companions to prevent such problems in the future. I also told her to do the same with her toes to help overcome what might be even more serious complaints caused by deep diving.

HOW TO STOP RINGING IN THE EARS

Many people have stopped ringing in their ears by working two reflex points located near the ears. First, open your mouth wide, and with your index finger, feel for a depression formed in front of the ears. This is a body warmer reflex. Then close your mouth and slightly work this reflex in a circular motion for about one minute. The other reflex can be located behind the ear, in a soft indented spot. See Diagram 15.

If these areas are very tender, you can work the reflex found on the hands or feet. The location of the ears will be found under the last two fingers or the last two toes. Refer to Diagrams 12 and 14.

THE REFLEX BUTTONS THAT HELP HEARING

It may not seem possible that by pressing a few reflexes a person who has been unable to hear for many years can suddenly regain his or her hearing. To these people, it is truly a very wonderful miracle.

Physicians familiar with the practice of reflexology have used this method for years to help the deaf hear. Osteopaths, chiropractors, and naturopathic doctors who have used this method of healing have had some very startling results.

Curing Deafness

In a previous book I told of many people who regained their hearing, some having been deaf for years. You, too, can use this simple method of reflexology to restore hearing to the deaf.

One simple method to use to bring back hearing, is to press and work the reflexes on the tip of the fourth finger. Pressing all around the top, sides, and beneath finger where it connects to palm of hand for several minutes at a time, doing this several times a day when possible. This will also relieve an earache.

The Hard Eraser Method

The hard eraser method has also been used successfully. You can use any sterile object, such as a hard eraser or whatever object will serve you best. Place this object in the space between the last tooth and the jaw, behind the wisdom tooth. You will be pressing on a reflex button that goes to the ear and is stimulated by a steady pressure. Bite down on this object for about five minutes at a time. Repeat this treatment several times a day.

The reflex comb is also very helpful in stimulating the ears. Press the teeth of the comb to the tips of all of the fingers and hold the pressure for about five minutes. See Photo 21.

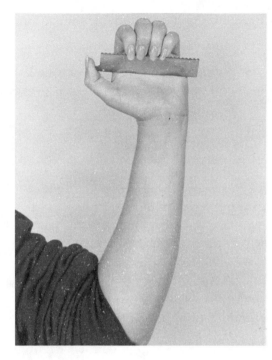

Photo 21: Position for holding reflex comb to alleviate pain in many parts of the body.

Reflexology for Better Hearing

One of my students told me of an almost deaf man who came to her for help. He could not hear very well even with a hearing aid. Without the hearing aid, he could hear practically nothing. After three or four visits to her for reflexology treatments, his hearing was greatly improved. She said the other day he told her that he could even hear the water running in a little creek located beside his home, something he had never heard before. His hearing gets better every day and he has thrown away his hearing aid.

> Dear Mrs. Carter,
>
> Just found out firsthand about reflexology and it worked for me. I couldn't hear correctly for more than forty years because my left ear was damaged during the war. Using reflex clamps on my left finger twice a day did the trick, and now I can even hear my wristwatch tick clearly.
>
> —Reverend S.H.

Energize your hearing by working the reflex to your cochlea, which is a snail-shell–shaped spiral cavity within your ear. You must energize the sensory nerve fibers so they can transmit sound to your brain. As you invigorate these sensory receptor cells, your hearing will become much sharper. Work the reflex buttons to your ears on your hands and feet.

PROTECT YOUR EARS

It is much easier to prevent a hearing problem than to cure one. Nerve damage caused by continued intense exposure to loud noise (for those who are employed in high-level-noise professions) must protect the ears with earplugs. Make sure you stimulate your auditory pathway by reflexing the pressure points to the ears, as well as around the ears.

REFLEXOLOGY HELPS RELEASE ELEVATION PRESSURE

When my daughter and her family were returning home from a trip in the mountains, where the elevation was nine thousand feet above sea level, they noticed a pressure in their ears. My daughter could not hear the radio very well and asked her family if they were experiencing the same discomfort. Her children were fine, but her husband said his ears were "plugged." They tried to yawn and chew gum to "open up" their ears, as this had worked for them in the past.

My daughter instinctively started pressing and working the reflex on the tip of her ring finger, pressing all around the top, sides, and beneath her ring and little fingers. Within two minutes, her ears were open and the pressure was released. She told her husband to do the same. He pressed the end of his ring finger, yawned and created a "pop"; he felt a slight draining in his ear and immediately felt better. He commented that it always amazes him how fast reflexology works. They noticed the radio seemed loud—their hearing was restored to normal, and they enjoyed the rest of their vacation—pain free.

CHAPTER 5

How to Use Reflex Pressure on the Tongue

The mouth and the tongue are not given enough consideration in most discussions of the healing forces of the body. All the food that we eat and all the liquids that we drink pass into the mouth and over the tongue. Many intricate, sensitive cells are exposed to all the elements as we drink hot and cold liquids. Alcoholic beverages and good foods and bad have to pass through this channel before we can nourish our bodies. Think of the importance of this organ as you study and learn to use the reflexes of the tongue and the mouth.

THE IMPORTANCE OF THE REFLEXES ON THE TONGUE

Most people don't realize that there are some very important reflexes in the mouth and the tongue. In fact, the tongue has reflex points that cover almost every part of the body. Everyone should have a tongue depressor and should use it every day to help keep in top condition. Take a tongue depressor or the handle of a spoon and press it on the tongue. See Photo 22. Turn it from side to side and press down. Feel the tender spots in various places on the tongue? By pressing the reflexes in the tongue you can overcome many types of pain and distress. Ten zones are in the tongue and they follow the pattern of the zones throughout the body. Note the zones in Diagram 16.

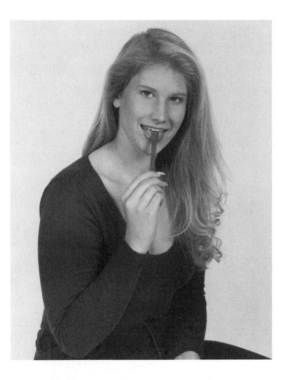

Photo 22: Shows reflex tongue probe ready to be used on the reflexes on the back of the tongue.

The reflexes in the center of the tongue correspond to the center of the body. So, as you press and stimulate the reflexes in the center of the tongue, you are sending the vital life force surging into all the glands, organs, and cells that are located in the center of the body. As you press on the reflexes on the right side of the tongue, you are stimulating all the glands and organs on the right side of the body. And when you press the reflexes on the left side of the tongue you are stimulating all the glands and organs on the left side of the body. When you find an extremely tender spot in a certain area of the tongue, check the zone chart to find just where there is malfunction in the body. Then press and hold this tender spot for a count of seven.

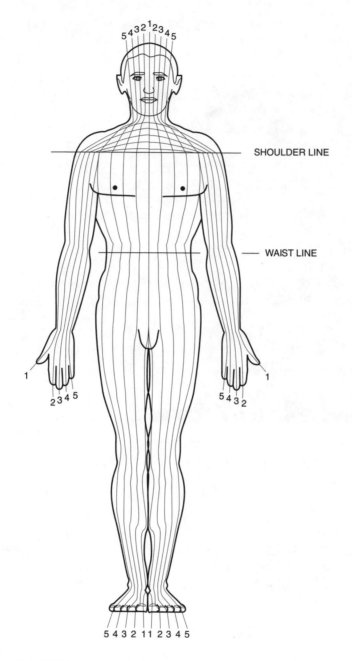

Diagram 16: *ZONE THERAPY:* Each numbered line represents the center of its respective zone on the body. These energy channels run longitudinally through the body.

CHECKING CORRESPONDING REFLEXES

Now, check the chart for other reflexes elsewhere on the body along this line, and when you press the ones corresponding to the reflex of the tongue, you will find that they are very tender also. Massage each button that shows tenderness. Remember that when there is tenderness in any part of the body, it is like a doorbell ringing to give you a message. The roller reflex massager is very helpful in locating tender buttons in various places on the body. This is explained more thoroughly in Chapter 36, on reflex devices.

Many people claim that they are never without their tongue depressor; they carry it with them in a sanitary plastic bag wherever they go.

The tongue reflexes are used to stop the pain of menstruation for women almost immediately. A pregnant woman should not press tongue reflexes since this seems to have a relaxing effect on the reproductive organs and might cause a miscarriage. Since it does relax and stop pain in various parts of the body, the tongue reflex might also prove beneficial to men who suffer from prostate trouble. I have no evidence on this, but always remember that wherever there is distress in any part of the body, reflexology can help, never harm.

There are also other reflexes in the mouth that help distressed parts of the body. Reflex buttons under the tongue and on the roof of the mouth bring relief from many ailments. By pressing the top of the mouth with a clean thumb, you will be able to stop coughs in a few minutes, if nothing else helps.

THE VALUE OF TONGUE PULLING

Grasping the tongue with a clean tissue or cloth and pulling out as far as possible (while holding the tongue up slightly to prevent cutting the under side of the tongue on the teeth) has several benefits. It can cure a sick voice and stop hiccups. Some life-saving clinics teach that pulling out the tongue relieves a choking person.

TONGUE BRUSHING

Do you realize how important it really is to clean the tongue? Asians have relied on tongue cleaning for centuries. It was a routine practice for the ancient Romans and is still used in the Orient as a natural method for freshening the breath, protecting the teeth, and killing harmful bacteria and germs.

Sylvia, a Chinese woman who was my second mother, taught me the importance of cleaning the tongue many years ago. She insisted that the tongue be scraped at least every morning and every night before retiring. This was more important to her than brushing the teeth. I don't remember what we used to scrape our tongues with at that time, but the habit has stayed with me and I have always brushed my tongue clean when I brush my teeth. Maybe that is why I have never had problems with my teeth.

The surface of the tongue is a breeding ground for bacteria. This germ-laden coating is a primary source of bad breath. Evidence has also been documented that plaque-forming streptococci counts increased ten times after a week of not cleaning the tongue.

The American Dental Association now encourages tongue cleaning. It has approved a tongue cleaner that is sold here in the United States called the Lila Tongue Cleaner. See Photo 23. If you are unable to find it on the market, you can purchase it from Stirling Enterprises, Cottage Grove, Oregon 97424.

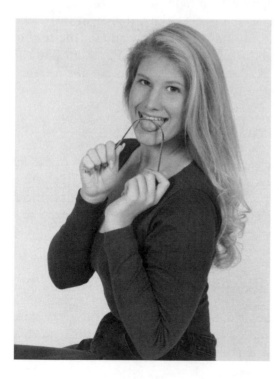

Photo 23: How to use the tongue scraper to cleanse the tongue.

CHAPTER 6

How Teeth Can Be Helped with Reflexology

I know of no pain more unbearable than a toothache. I am lucky to have had very few problems with my teeth. The ones that I have suffered from have been caused by dentists. I had been exposed to severe cold and had gotten neuralgia in the nerves in my face, which was very painful. I thought that the pain might be caused by a tooth, but I couldn't get to see a dentist for several days. I knew that reflexology could help stop the pain, so I used clamps on my fingers off and on until I could see the dentist. This deadened the pain, and I don't know what made me keep my appointment with the dentist, but I did. When I got into the chair, he could not find anything wrong with my teeth. He was very concerned for my comfort, so he decided that he should pull one of my teeth even though the X-ray showed it to be perfect, as were all my teeth. I don't know why, but I let him pull it. I think that when we get in front of a doctor or a dentist we become hypnotized in some way. That is the only tooth that I have ever lost.

AN EFFECTIVE TOOTHPASTE

A dentist I went to many years ago for a mouth infection told me that I had perfect teeth and gums and asked what I used for toothpaste. I told him that I had used salt and soda all my life. He said that was the reason that I had hard, healthy gums and teeth. The glycerine used in toothpastes, he said, tended to soften the gums. When I mentioned this to certain other dentists, they made fun of me and said that it had nothing to do with my hard gums and perfect teeth.

Now we are told by Dr. Paul Keyes, clinical investigator at the National Institute of Dental Research, that gum disease can be prevented simply by brushing with *salt*. He says that if you have high blood pressure and are not supposed to use table salt, you can substitute Epsom salt.

How I Make My Tooth Cleaner

I use a salt shaker with large holes. In this, I put equal parts of salt and soda and two or three beans to keep the mixture from caking into hard lumps. I sprinkle a small amount of this in my hand and apply it with a dampened toothbrush. You will never have a fresher-feeling mouth or whiter teeth. The salt cleans and hardens the gums and the soda polishes the teeth "harmlessly." After brushing, rinse with hydrogen peroxide to whiten your teeth and clean your gums. Peroxide kills germs, which helps your mouth stay healthy. My children had perfect teeth until they left home and turned to the use of toothpastes and the consumption of sugared products such as candies and soft drinks. Maybe if they had kept using the salt and soda, the sugared products would have been less harmful to their teeth.

Dr. Keyes stresses that this program would be very beneficial for anyone with incipient pyorrhea. About 95 percent of the population suffers from some form of gum disease, from simple to advanced.

If you want fewer tooth problems, try the methods that I have described in this book. They will work wonders for you.

Stopping a Toothache

To stop the pain of toothache, clamp down near the ends of the fingers. Check the meridian lines and press the fingers of the hand that is on the same side as the sore tooth. See Diagram 16. Follow the line that would go through the aching tooth down to the fingers on this same line, and put pressure on the fingers to which this line leads. This will anesthetize this area, and you will be free from pain. If you do not have clamps or rubber bands, hold pressure on the fingers with the teeth until the pain subsides. You will probably have to do this every fifteen to twenty minutes to keep the area deadened and free from pain until you can see a dentist.

Toothache Stopped with a Comb and Finger Clamp

At a dinner dance one evening, the hostess told me she had an intolerable toothache. Since she had been a patient of mine, she was hoping I could help her. We went to the dressing room and I asked her for a comb. Since the tooth that was aching was on the left side, I began pressing her fingers on the left hand. I found some very tender spots on the inside of the thumb and index finger. Commencing with light pressure on these sensitive areas, I gradually increased the pressure on the comb while we talked of subjects pertaining to the party for about ten minutes. I asked how her tooth was, and she was astonished to find that the pain had left while we were talking. She enjoyed the rest of the evening without any further pain. I told her that she would be wise to use clamps on her fingers once in a while (and also a comb) until she could see her dentist. She said that she would never be without them again.

An Embarrassing Situation Avoided

One evening, my husband was at a lodge meeting. A man sitting next to him complained of a terrible toothache and said he thought he would have to leave because of the pain. He was embarrassed as he was an important speaker for the evening. My husband told him to squeeze firmly on the joint of the middle finger, since the tooth that was causing him the pain was in the third meridian line of the body. The man knew that my husband was well informed on the healing methods of reflexology, so he followed the advice without any argument. He was amazed and very grateful to find that the tooth had completely stopped hurting by the time he was called on to give his talk. Later, when he thanked my husband for saving him from an embarrassing situation, he confessed that he was so amazed at the sudden relief from the toothache, that he nearly forgot his speech.

Reflex Percussion of the Gums

Now let us reflex massage the buttons near the roots of the teeth. Press all your fingers into your cheeks and feel for the roots of the upper teeth. Starting in front of the ears, work the fingers slowly toward the center of the face until you are pressing under the nose. Hold pressure on each of these buttons for about three seconds each. You may find some tender spots as your fingers travel over this area. When you do, hold pressure on this sore button a little longer, or go back and hold the pressure again later.

Now go to the roots of the lower teeth. Place all the fingers along the line of the jawbone starting at the ears. As you press in, you will feel the roots of the lower teeth. Work your fingers along this area as you did on the roots of the upper teeth, pressing and massaging until you are working on the roots of the front teeth at the chin. See Photo 24. You stimulate the small and large intestine as well as the stomach meridians when you drum these areas with the finger. While your fingers are in this position, place the thumbs under the chin and massage this area toward the chin. This helps reduce a double chin. See Photo 25.

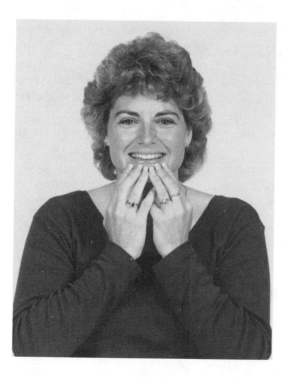

Photo 24: Position for pressing roots to lower teeth.

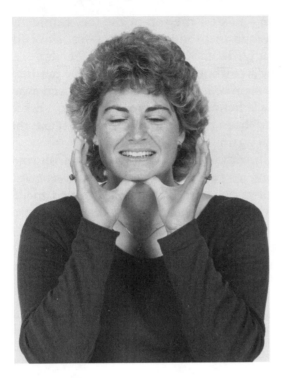

Photo 25: Pressing lymph nodes under the chin with the thumbs to make this area soft and pliable to increase energy and the flow of hormones for better skin and fewer wrinkles.

A Test of Reflexology

A friend came to me one day suffering with a terrible toothache. We were in the mountains and there was no one to help her but me. She begged me to take her to a dentist, so I dropped everything and drove about twenty miles to a small country town where we found the dentist's office closed. We contacted the dentist and talked him into helping my friend, though he was against doing anything since she was pregnant and the tooth was ulcerated. He finally did pull the tooth after deadening it. When we were about halfway home, my friend started to cry and complained that she still had a toothache. I took her back to the dentist, but he refused to do anything for the other tooth, which was also badly abscessed. He told us that it would be too dangerous in her condition.

On the way home, I told her we would try reflexology on it. She was willing to try anything. As soon as we arrived home, I had her sit in a chair and give me her bare feet. I started to press on a big toe, and upon finding a very sore reflex on the top of the toe, I immediately used the press-and-massage method. In just seconds, she said, "Oh, it's getting better already." In about half an hour, the pain had completely subsided, and she went home promising to have her husband take her to a dentist as soon as he came home. We moved away soon after that, so I did not see her for several months. When I asked about her teeth, she said she hadn't gone to a dentist because the tooth had never bothered her again.

Don't forget to eat foods with plenty of calcium to nourish your teeth. A dentist tells of treating his patients with calcium and relieving them of all kinds of tooth diseases. The teeth actually healed themselves when nature was called in to do her work and was given the material to work with.

With a little knowledge about the tooth and its needs and how to give nature a helping hand, you may be able to keep your teeth for as long as you live.

CHAPTER 7

How to Use Reflexology on the Eyes for Better Eyesight

Our eyes are truly a precious gift from God. Only those who have been denied the gift of sight or those who have lost it truly understand its importance.

Reflexology has helped many in different stages of blindness. It can do no harm and it is always of some benefit even if it fails to give a person perfect eyesight. Reflex massage always relaxes, no matter what one is using it for, and that in itself is good.

I hope that I can bring a new understanding to you who are having eye problems and that you will give reflex massage a chance to prove to you that it really can help. You can also bring more beauty to the eyes by using reflex massage as directed.

STIMULATING THE KIDNEYS TO STRENGTHEN YOUR EYES

Two of the most important organs affecting normal functioning of the eyes are the kidneys.

To stimulate the kidneys, massage the reflexes in the center of the feet and also the hands. See Diagrams 3 and 5. See Diagrams 7 and 8 for body reflexes to the kidneys and work on these to help stimulate the eyes.

Now turn to the reflexes of the eyes themselves. In my previous books on foot reflexology and hand reflexology, I taught you to massage the reflexes just under the two toes next to the big toes where they fasten to the foot, doing this massage on both feet. Use the same massage on the two fingers next to the thumb. If these are tender, the reflexes are in need of massage to break loose certain blockages affecting the normal function of the eyes.

MASSAGING EYE REFLEXES FOR BETTER EYESIGHT

Now we turn to massage of the reflexes near the eyes for correction of many eye problems. The following method was worked out and used successfully by Therese Pfrimmer. If there is tightness of muscles around the eyes, they may pull on the eyeball, distort its shape, and cut off circulation, causing near- and far-sightedness. Tight eyelid muscles sometimes cause friction on the eyeball that can lead to the formation of cataracts. If the eye muscles in the back of the eye are tight, the drainage ducts will be squeezed shut and won't empty properly. This can cause a buildup of fluid resulting in glaucoma.

To loosen the eye muscles, take your middle fingers and massage along the reflexes underneath both eyes. See Photo 26. Press in as you go across and feel for tight muscles. When you find that a muscle is tight, you will also probably find a hard spot or feel the muscles snap under your fingers. When you stimulate the reflexes to the eyes you immediately give renewed energy and life to your eyes. Don't do this very often at first. When you overstimulate the eyes, it can give you a terrible headache. I suggest that you do this only once the first day; then increase as you feel that you can, without any overstimulation. This holds true for the other eye reflex massages and also for the eye exercises I will give you later.

Move to the bones on top of the eyes and repeat the procedure. It may be easier to use the thumbs for this position. Work across the muscles and not with them when you do this massage.

Take your middle finger or thumb and work across the muscles on top of the nose starting deep in the eye socket. You will probably find this very tender, but remember our motto, "If it hurts, rub it out." Do this to both eyes; then go across the muscles on the forehead just above the eyebrows. If you feel a hard core or a tight band,

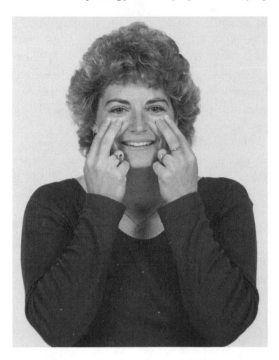

Photo 26: How to press the reflexes to the kidneys and adrenal glands for better eyesight.

you will know that you have found a tight muscle that may restrict the natural flow of electrical energy by way of the reflexes. It will probably be quite tender because the circulation of the vital life line is being blocked by these hard or tender areas.

Massaging these reflexes around the eyes can also help correct protruding eyes, eyes that hurt or are sensitive to light, and slanted eyes caused by muscle tension.

Massaging and tapping on the head can also help stimulate new life to the eyes. See Chapter 3, on the head.

AN ALL-NATURAL EYE WASH

Another method of helping the eyes get back to normal is using honey. Just put a drop or so of honey in the eyes and in a very short time you will notice an improvement. It burns like fire at first, but only for a few seconds; the tears soon wash it out. I had a bad case of night blindness once. A lot of people were putting honey in their eyes, so I decided I would try it. A very short time after using honey, I was forced to drive home after dark. I had driven several miles when I realized that I could see just as well as I could in the daytime. That was several years ago, and I can still see well at night. I only used the honey about ten days, and then got busy and forgot to use it again.

PALMING TO HELP THE EYES

Another thing that helps eyes is palming them. One man actually saved his eyesight by palming his eyes several times a day. To do this, put the palms of your hands on each eye, crossing the fingers over each other. Now, adjust them so that no light gets through. Keep your eyes open. Hold them in this position for a few minutes, being sure that you are looking into complete darkness. This is also very relaxing to the whole nervous system. Do it several times a day if you wish.

HOW TO RELIEVE EYESTRAIN

Improving the blood circulation to the forehead and temples will relieve eyestrain. Use the knuckles or tips, of your middle fingers, and with a light, circular motion work the temples, located on each side of the forehead at the outer edge of each eyebrow.

Vitamins A and C are important to good eyesight. I found a juicer to be a wonderful investment. It is hard to eat enough fresh salads to equal all the natural nutrition needed for good vision.

Adjust the Foot to Straighten the Eye

My brother always had a problem with his left foot. It turned in and he would stumble over it with the right foot and fall frequently.

When my son was born, he had the same problem. I noticed his left eye turned in also. I made some lifts for his shoe to straighten his foot out, and when his foot straightened out, so did his eye.

EYE EXERCISES

Here are some eye exercises that are very helpful in strengthening the eyes. Years ago when my parents were prospecting in the Sierra Mountains, we met a doctor who taught us these exercises. I feel that because of them we didn't have to wear glasses for many years, and if we had kept up with the exercises we probably would never have had to wear them. I had my daughter do them after she suffered bad eye-strain that caused her to blink her eyes repeatedly. Her eyes returned to normal in just a few days.

Sit down where you can place a center mark on a wall directly in front of you, level with the eyes. A very tiny spot is all that is needed. The bathroom can be an excellent place to do this since it only takes a few minutes and it is one place where you aren't disturbed. You might want to place a mark in each bathroom if you have a large family and teach them all how to use this eye-strengthening exercise. It can cut down on doctor bills.

You are now sitting with the spot directly in front of you. *Very slowly* turn your eyes to the left as far as you can without moving the head and *very slowly* bring them back to the center spot. Repeat the procedure looking to the right and back. From the center spot, lift the eyes up as far as possible. Be sure to keep the head straight and always bring the eyes back to the marked spot before doing the next movement. Do this only once the first few days. If you overdo these exercises, you will get one of the worst headaches you have ever had. This proves how very potent they are. Increase the number of repetitions every few days until you can do them ten times a day.

After the eyes have become used to this exercise, start to roll the eyes. Turn the eyes to the left as far as you can, then start to roll them up *slowly*. Roll them up and to the right and then down and on around till you have them back on the left side. Do this only once a day to start. Keep the head straight and do this exercise *very slowly*. You may gradually work this up to ten times a day.

How many times do you look a long distance away? Practice looking at great distances and then at something very close. These muscles need exercise, too.

You should be able to develop perfect eyesight by using one or several of the methods that I have given you.

Teach these eye-strengthening techniques to your children, and they may be blessed with perfect eyesight the rest of their lives.

Using Clamps on the Eyebrows

Dear Mrs. Carter,

I have been experimenting with reflexology clamps and they truly work miracles on many parts of the body besides the fingers and toes. By placing them on the lips you can stimulate the circulation to the sagging muscles around the mouth. By putting them on the eyebrows, they not only stimulate circulation to the wrinkles around the eyes but strengthen the eyes as well. When I showed these clamps to a doctor, he immediately put one on his eyebrow, instead of his finger, before I had time to tell him how to use them.

He is very enthusiastic about the possibilities of stimulating the healing life force in many parts of the body. He says by using this form of pressure on any part of the body it will increase the productivity of healing by added circulation.

—C.S.

CHAPTER 8

How Reflexology Stimulates the Endocrine Glands

The endocrine glands have no ducts and secrete their hormones directly into the bloodstream. If you will look at Diagram 2, you will see the most important endocrine glands as they are located in the body. To those who study Hindu teachings, these are referred to as *chakras* or energy centers.

The pituitary gland is located near the center of the head, along with the pineal gland. The thyroid and parathyroids are near the larynx at the base of the neck. The thymus is located in the chest area. The pancreas is lower in the body under the stomach and above the adrenals (or superadrenals), which are like little caps on the kidneys. Then, we move down to the lower area of the body to the gonads or sex glands (testes and ovaries) of men and women.

THE IMPORTANCE OF THE ENDOCRINE GLANDS

All these glands supplement and interact with each other. Their normal development and functions are of great importance to the well-being of every individual. The hormones that they secrete are responsible for the differences between a very small person and a very large person, a genius and someone of low intelligence, a happy or a cheerless individual. They control what we are—our energy, activity, radiance, and stability as well as the vitalization of the life processes. Their influence is pervasive in all that we do and are. They are responsible for determining the forms of our bodies and the workings of our minds.

THE PITUITARY GLAND

A person who is relaxed and generally happy, without any frustrations, is sure to possess a normal, healthy pituitary gland. If you are not all of these, then you should check the reflexes to the pituitary gland, located in the center of the pad of the big toe and the center of the pad on the thumb. See Diagram 2. You will also find reflex buttons to the pituitary located on the forehead. See Diagram 12. This gland also helps prevent an excessive accumulation of fat. If you are trying to lose weight, there is reason for you to give the reflexes to the pituitary gland special attention.

In a study conducted several years ago, it was found that disobedience, bullying, moroseness, and many types of child delinquency were caused by a faulty pituitary gland.

The pituitary gland is likened to a first violin in keeping the body in harmony. If it is out of tune, the whole body is out of harmony, and no one can feel in top condition if his or her glands are not *all* in tune with each other. This gland is responsible for proper growth of our body glands and organs, including normal sexual development.

The pituitary gland is one of the controllers of growth, so if you are concerned about the growth rate of your child, be sure to massage the reflexes to your child's pituitary gland. This will stabilize the growth rate to normal whether your child is growing too fast or too slowly. If this area is tender, it should be massaged often. Teach children to massage this special button for themselves to help keep their growth rate normal and learn to use it in helping other malfunctioning areas as well.

THE PINEAL GLAND

The pineal gland controls the development of the other glands, keeping them in their proper range. The malfunction of the pineal gland influences the sex glands, causing the premature development of the entire system. This gland keeps the normal activity of the endocrine system harmonious and effective.

THE THYROID GLAND

The degree of thyroid activity makes a person either dull or alert, animated or depressed, quick or slow. The development and activity of the sex glands also depend on a normal and healthy thyroid.

The important reflexes for the thyroid gland are located in the hands and the feet. Find the reflex to the thyroid gland just under the large pads near the big toes. These will be on both feet. The reflexes on the left foot stimulate the thyroid on the left side and those on the right foot stimulate the thyroid on the right side. This is also true of the reflexes on the hands near the thumbs. See Diagram 2.

Use the thumb, the fingers, or a reflex massager and press in under the foot pads and hand pads. See Photos 27 and 28. You will probably find some very tender buttons in this area, so you must massage the soreness out—but not all at once. Send these healing life forces to the malfunctioning thyroid a little at a time until it once again returns to a normal and healthy working order.

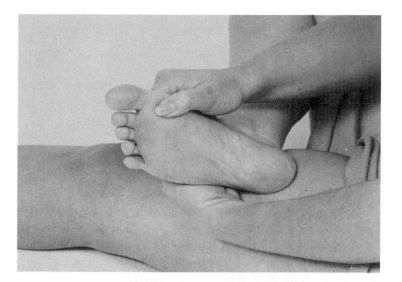

Photo 27: Position for massaging the reflexes in the feet to stimulate the thyroid gland.

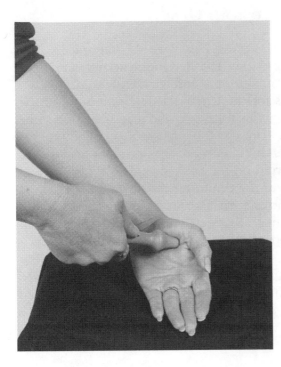

Photo 28: Using reflex hand probe to massage many important reflexes to the body, including the reflexes to the thyroid.

Now, we will look to the reflexes for the thyroids in other parts of the body. As you look at Diagrams 2 and 10, you can see that the thyroids are located on each side of the throat, and in Diagrams 7 and 8 you will see that the reflexes to the thyroids are located on the neck. See Photo 29 to learn the positions for massaging the reflexes to these important glands. Place the fingers on one side of the throat and the thumb on the opposite side. See Photo 30. Now, starting close to the jaw, use a gentle rolling motion with the fingers. You need not press hard here—we do not want to bruise the thyroids in any way. Use this rolling massage, working down to the collarbone. Now use this same rolling massage and work back up to the jaw bone. Now change hands so that the thumb will be on the opposite side of the throat and again go through the same procedure, massaging down to the collarbone and back up to the jaw. I would advise you to go slowly and do this once or twice the first day. Increase the amount of time you spend doing this massage gradually as you feel it is necessary.

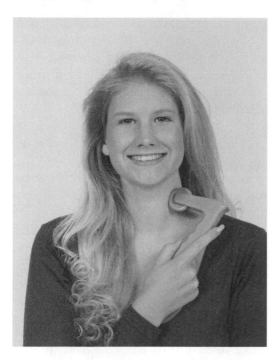

Photo 29: Using the reflex roller massager to stimulate the thyroid gland.

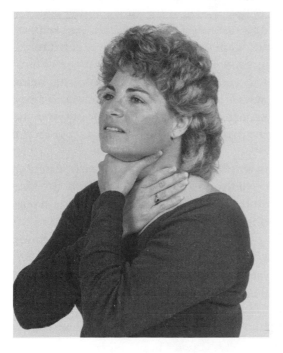

Photo 30: Position for massaging reflexes in the neck and throat to stimulate thyroid and other hormone-producing glands.

Look at Photo 25 to see how the thumbs are hooked under the jaw bone and chin. This should be done with a gentle pressing motion two or three times on each side. These particular reflexes will, when stimulated by massage as I showed you, develop beautifully firm and smooth skin, of which I will tell you more in Chapter 34, on beauty. It is also said to keep the hair from turning gray.

Let us look at one more reflex to the thyroid gland. If you try to find the very center of the top of your head, you find a sensitive reflex to the thyroid glands. See Photo 16. This, of course, will stimulate parathyroids also. It should be located on a straight line from the front of the ears. Feel for it—every head is shaped differently. Now, place the middle fingers of both hands on this reflex and hold it for a few seconds, then release. Do this three times—not any more than that at first. The middle finger of one hand may be used if you feel you could get better results.

THE PARATHYROIDS

The parathyroids, four tiny bead-sized glands embedded in the surface of the thyroid, carry an enormous responsibility in keeping your body functioning in perfect order. The normal functioning of these glands results in poise and tranquility. They influence the stability within your body and the maintenance of its metabolic equilibrium by controlling the distribution and activity of calcium and phosphorus in the system. These represent a certain polarity—phosphorus being connected with the nervous system, calcium with the skeletal. I hope you will recognize the dynamic factor we have on one side and the static one on the other. The parathyroids maintain a balance between them.

The reflexes to these all-important little glands are located in about the same area as the thyroid reflexes on the hands and the feet, but you will have to press in more deeply for the parathyroids. From what I have just told you about these glands, you will recognize how important it is to keep them functioning in perfect order at all times. You will probably have to use the little hand massager (see Photo 28) to reach in deeply enough to stimulate them with renewed electric life force. As you massage the reflexes on the hands and the feet, you may find them extremely tender. You must give them special attention until they are no longer so painful when pressed with the massager.

Some people always find a certain amount of tenderness in the reflexes in the parathyroid areas, so you should massage them each time you give yourself a treatment.

THE THYMUS GLAND

The thymus is a pinkish-gray, two-lobed organ located high in the chest behind the breast bone. See Diagrams 7 and 8.

There has been a misconception concerning the role the thymus plays in our overall health. It was believed that the thymus diminishes in size as we reach puberty and becomes useless, which has been proven to be untrue by Dr. John Diamond. In his book, *Your Body Doesn't Lie,* he tells us, "The thymus can be considered to be a true endocrine gland—that is, an organ that secretes a hormone into the bloodstream to be carried to another part of the body where it will have its effect."

Dr. Diamond tells us, "The evidence accumulated over the last twenty years on the thymus gland's role in immunology is overwhelming. In a human being or an animal in which the thymus gland has been removed or destroyed, there is a loss of effectiveness of the immune mechanisms of the body that guard against infection and cancerous growths."

People become more susceptible to all types of diseases as they become older because they let the thymus become weak. It may be one of the most important glands in your body; it is the seat of life energy. When the thymus becomes weak you lose energy.

The thymus gland is involved with the strength of muscular contraction and can be tested by using applied kinesiology (which can also be used to overcome stress or determine the cause of it).

The thymus is involved in the flow of lymph throughout the body. The lymphatic system drains foreign matter, cellular debris, and toxins from the cells and carries them to the bloodstream for disposal.

The Thymus Is the Home Base of Energy

The thymus gland monitors and regulates energy flow throughout the body energy system, initiating instantaneous corrections to overcome imbalances as they occur so as to achieve a rebalancing and harmony of body energy.

Dr. Diamond also tells us, "The thymus gland is the link between mind and body, being the first organ to be affected by mental attitudes and stress!"

We learn that many things in life can so deplete our energy that they cause all the muscles in our body to become weak; these include the wrong kind of food, sugar, and chemical additives. Sitting on a soft seat, especially in a car, can cause us to be less mentally alert by weakening our minds and our muscles. Just being near certain people can drain our energy. Negative thoughts, loud or inharmonious music, and certain colors can also deplete our energy, as does continual stress.

How to Reactivate the Thymus

Let me tell you how you can use reflexology to reactivate the energy in the thymus gland quickly, thus strengthening the weakened muscles in the body. See Diagrams 2, 7, and 8 and note the location of the thymus gland in the chest. If you take the ends of the fingers and tap the chest several times over the thymus gland, you will stimulate the gland so that it will send energy quickly to all the body muscles.

An inconspicuous way to return the thymus to quick normal activity is to press a reflex to the thymus that is located in the roof of your mouth, just in front of the teeth. Press this reflex with the tip of your tongue.

How to Test with Kinesiology

Let us test the power of the thymus over the weakening and the strengthening of the muscles by the short and simple method of kinesiology. You will require a partner. Have the partner stand in front of you with his or her left arm held out parallel to the floor while his right arm is relaxed at his side. Now, standing in front of the person, place your left hand on his shoulder to steady him. Tell him that you are going to press down the arm he is holding out straight and that he is to resist. Place your right hand on his arm just above the wrist. Press his arm firmly, just enough to test the strength of his muscles. This is not a contest of strength. If the arm is weak, have him tap the thymus reflex on his chest or press the thymus reflex in front of the teeth in the center of the roof of his mouth with the tip of his tongue, and test again. The muscles should now be strong.

While his muscles are strong, have him put a little sugar in his mouth, think of an unpleasant situation, listen to inharmonious music or sounds, or perform another stress-causing action before he tries the test again. If you are doing this correctly, the muscles will have become very weak and he will not be able to resist a slight pressure. Think of all the muscles in your body losing energy and becoming weak so quickly from such a slight cause of stress. Do you wonder why so many people are upset and ill without knowing why?

TESTING FOR POSITIVE LIFE ENERGY

Now let us turn to positive things that will reactivate your thymus into raising your life energy rather than depleting it.

There are many more positive ways to reactivate the thymus than there are negative, so let us learn a few of them. Let us first turn to nature.

Dr. Diamond tells us, "The normal position of the tongue is to keep the tip against the centering reflex in the roof of the mouth at all times. In this position the entire body is tonified through the relationship between the centering reflex button and the body energy system and the life energy." Every time you smile you are also stimulating the reflexes to the thymus gland. Smiling is a body energizer, so think positive thoughts; keep your mind on happy thoughts at all times; feel the vibrations of love for all things beautiful. Sit straight; listen to good music; eat only good natural food. Be thankful and joyful in all things. Do the words "love, faith, hope, and charity" have a deeper meaning for you? Were these words given to us as body energizers as well as for spiritual upliftment?

How to Massage Other Reflexes to the Thymus Gland

Look to another reflex to the thymus that is located in the bottom of the feet. See Diagram 2. You will also find this thymus reflex in the hands. See Photos 31 and 32 for use of the reflex roller and the magic reflex massager to stimulate all reflexes to most of the body located in the hands.

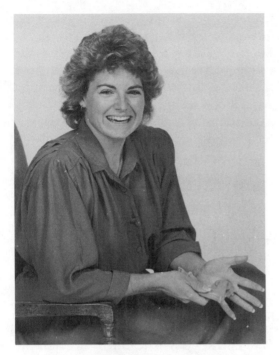

Photo 31: Shows an easy method of using the reflex roller to massage the reflexes in the hand. Laughter will stimulate your lymphatic system and improve your health.

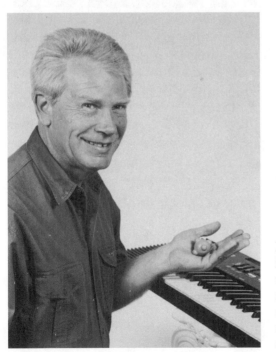

Photo 32: Organ teacher instructs students on how to use the magic reflex massager before playing a musical instrument. It relaxes the fingers and stimulates the mind.

You will also find reflexes to the thymus located in the head. See Diagram 16 on page 54. Anything on the center line will help stimulate the thymus gland.

I hope you are now more conscious of the importance of the thymus. Square dancers live long healthy lives. They stimulate the thymus with good music, laughter, and fun in their dances. Keep smiling and laughing at all times, thus reactivating your thymus gland into raising your life energy instead of depleting it with negative vibrations.

THE PANCREAS

The pancreas is a large gland located in the midsection of the body. It is really two glands: the major part of the pancreas secretes digestive juices, and other cells within the pancreas secrete the hormone insulin, which maintains the body's sugar level.

In Diagrams 2, 7, and 9, see the position of the pancreas in relation to other abdominal organs and glands in the body. Notice in Diagram 7 how the reflex to the pancreas is located in about the same position as the reflex to the spleen as shown in Diagram 8. When we massage the reflexes in this area, we will be sending the stimulation of electrical energy into both glands simultaneously.

We will also be stimulating these and other glands as we massage the reflexes to the pancreas located in the hands and the feet. Start on the left foot, and with your thumb or whatever you use to massage the reflexes, start just below the pad of the big toe where we found the thyroid reflexes. See Diagram 2 and Photo 33. With a rolling method, massage clear across the foot, searching for sore buttons. Remember, whenever you find a button that is sensitive to the touch, no matter where it is located (unless it is a bruise or a swollen area), either apply pressure or use the massage technique.

Now turn to the reflex in the hands. Using the thumb or a device with a massaging, pressing motion, massage completely across the center of the opposite hand. Work toward the web between the thumb and the forefinger, searching for tender buttons as you go across the hand. See Diagram 2 and Photos 34 and "C" on page 109. Do this to both hands two or three times; then pinch and massage this web in both hands, working clear up between the bones of the thumb and the finger. See Diagrams 6A, 6D, and 6E and Photos 35 and 36. This seems to be a "hot spot" for the reflexes to many parts of the body, so don't neglect it. It aids in the flow of the vital electrical life force, no matter the part of the body to which we are attempting to clear the channels.

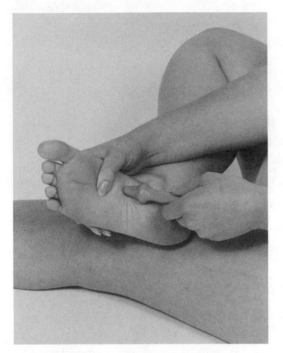

Photo 33: Shows use of reflex probe to work reflexes to stomach area, (thumb is on reflex to adrenal gland.)

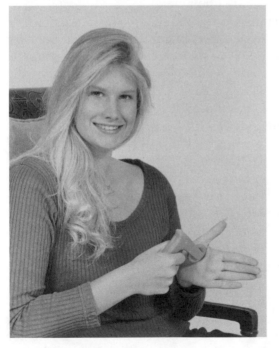

Photo 34: Massaging reflexes in the hand to stimulate many parts of the body.

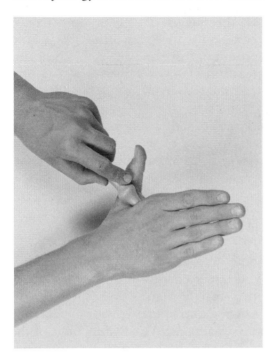

Photo 35: Using reflex hand probe to stimulate many parts of the body—great for pain relief, insomnia, and anxiety.

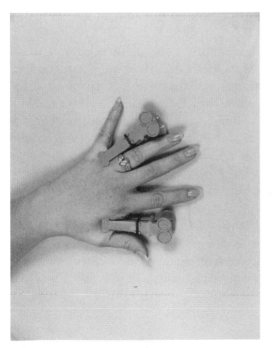

Photo 36: Shows reflex clamps used on the webs of the hands, which benefits many parts of the body.

Turn to Diagram 7. With the fingers of one or both hands, whichever seems to give the best results, press into the area a little below the ribs. Hold to a slow count of three and release. Repeat this three times. Because the pancreas spreads over a large area, you may move the fingers an inch toward the center of the body and repeat almost all the way across.

See Diagram 12 for the location of the reflex buttons on the head and above the lips. There are also reflex buttons in the ears which are not shown, but when you massage the ears you will be stimulating the reflexes to the pancreas.

THE ADRENAL GLANDS

Your glands control every minute of your life from cradle to grave. The adrenal glands promote your inner energy—the drive to action. The adrenal glands consist of two small triangular bodies lying above and in front of the kidneys. The cortex, the outer part of the adrenal, produces three types of hormones that control many functions of the body, including water and salt balances, and carbohydrate, protein, and fat metabolism. The inner part of the adrenal produces the hormone adrenalin, which instantly prepares the body to react to an emergency.

To stimulate the adrenal glands and keep them in perfect working order, first turn to the reflexes located in the hands and the feet. By looking at Diagram 11, you can see that the adrenals are located on top of the kidneys, so the reflexes will be just a little above the kidney reflexes in the center of the hands and a little above the center in the feet. See Diagrams 3 and 5. If this area is tender at all, the adrenals are probably telling you that they are not getting a full supply of energy. Somewhere in the lines the power is getting short-circuited, so you will have to push a few buttons to correct the power shortage. Press and massage these buttons with the thumbs or a reflex massager several times, but be aware that they lie so close to the kidneys that you cannot help but massage the reflexes to the kidneys as well as the adrenal glands. We do not want to overmassage the kidney reflexes in the beginning, so, to start, only massage the adrenals for about five seconds.

Look at Diagram 12 for the location of the adrenal reflexes on the head and Diagrams 7 and 8 for body location. You will see also the kidney reflexes; you have learned that when you massage the reflexes to the kidneys, the adrenals are also helped. Press and hold gently on body reflexes shown in Diagrams 7 and 8.

THE GONADS—THE SEX GLANDS

The gonads—in men the testes, in women the ovaries—are located in the lower part of the body. The pituitary gland produces the hormone that activates the gonads to begin puberty.

The endocrine glands are critical to proper functioning, and reflexology can normalize endocrine-related problems that may occur. Our glandular system is the transmitter of life forces that are transformed into functions throughout the body. By using reflex massage on the reflexes to these glands, we help stimulate the whole body. See Photo 37.

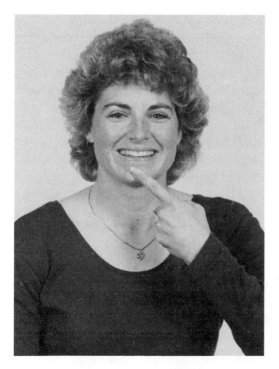

Photo 37: Position for massaging the reflexes to the gonads, which gives warmth to the system, sparkling eyes, and luminosity.

Look at Diagram 2 to find where the gonads are located in the body. In Diagram 4 you will find the reflexes to the gonads located near the ankles on the outside of the feet—the testes for the men and the ovaries for the women. On the inside of the feet (near the ankles) are the reflexes for the uterus in the women and for the penis in the men. This will also be an area to massage for prostate trouble. For the gonad reflexes, you will also pinch and massage the cord up the back of the leg, the Achilles tendon.

On the hands, find the reflexes that involve the wrists. Search here for tender buttons on all parts of the wrist. When you find a sore button, massage it out. See Diagram 2 and Photo 38.

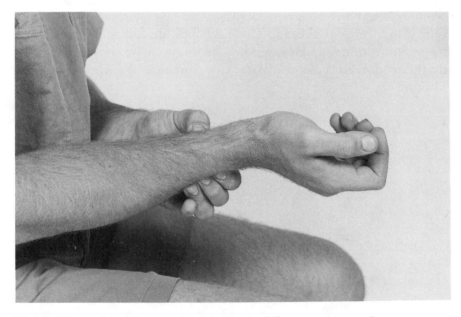

Photo 38: Position for stopping nausea and for massaging reflexes to reproductive organs and other parts of the body.

There are more reflexes that will help the gonads, which I will explain more fully in the chapter on sex and its related problems.

Complete Recovery Through Reflex Massage

While giving a seminar in Alaska on reflexology, I met a very sick woman. By her color I knew there was something seriously wrong with her. She was a secretary and told me that she had been subjected to insecticide spray poisoning while at work, due to the many insects and doctors did not know what to do for her. She suffered most of the time without knowing how to get help. I told her I might be able to help her, as the poison was probably in the lymphatic system. She was willing to try anything to be well again.

I massaged her whole body for two hours at a time, pressing and pulling with my fingertips. I had to extend my stay for a few days, but it was worth it because she recovered almost completely before I left. Now she uses reflexology on herself to help free her body of this accumulation of toxic poison.

CHAPTER 9

How Reflexology Strengthens an Ailing Heart and Blood Circulation

Everyone should be more aware of the heart and how to massage the reflexes to keep it in perfect working condition. All life processes are rhythmic alterations of tension and release of tension. Blood moves from the lungs where it is oxygenated to the small intestines where it begins to give up oxygen, making these two opposite organs, lungs and the small intestines, the poles. The heart beats as the flow of oxygenated and deoxygenated blood moves through it, creating tension and release of tension. Ancient traditional medicine declares, "The meridian of the heart rules the arteries between the lungs and the small intestines and the lung rules over the heart."

The heart controls the mind. If the heart is weak, like a ruler without power, it invites revolt. When a multitude of body areas are malfunctioning and the problem cannot be pinpointed, it means that the electric life force is not flowing freely through the meridian channels. See Diagram 16.

A Massage to Help the Heart

Dear Mrs. Carter,

I am seventy-seven years young, and this morning I sure thought my heart was giving up. I massaged the reflexes for a half-hour and, thank God, I am feeling better.

Kindly inform me if I can find a doctor who practices reflex-ology in my vicinity. Thank you and God bless you and yours.

—Mrs. K.P.

REFLEX POINTS TO HELP
THE HEART AND CIRCULATION

No matter what your heart problems might be, reflexology can help. Remember that a malfunctioning heart is usually caused by a problem in some other area of the body.

We are all aware that the heart is the pumping station that keeps the body functioning. Like the pump of a well, if the heart slows down, the circulation of the life lines slows down. The fluid, be it water or blood, will not do a complete job of circulating to all areas needed; thus, certain areas that are denied full circulation become weak, and deterioration sets in.

The heart is a strong muscle. By pressing certain reflex buttons located on the feet and the hands and several places on the body, this great muscle can be kept at top efficiency. If there is a malfunction, you can help it to function normally by pressing and massaging the heart reflex buttons.

See the reflex buttons near the spine on Diagram 18B, in Chapter 27. To help an ailing heart you can use these reflexes, but you will need someone else to help you. Just have your partner find the tender spots and press or massage until soreness is relieved. If the spine is out of adjustment, your chiropractor can help put it into place. Be sure to go to a reputable chiropractor.

DEEP MUSCLE THERAPY FOR THE HEART

Deep muscle therapy, according to Mrs. Pfrimmer, also helps the heart. She claims that deep muscle massage has helped all kinds of heart problems. So along with your diet for the heart and reflex mas-saging of the heart reflexes, you should help the heart by loosening the muscles, by going deeper than the reflexes and massaging the deep muscles that could be causing lack of circulation to the heart.

First work on the muscles of the left arm as this is a major source of blood to the heart. Start massaging these muscles at the wrist of the left arm. You are not massaging reflex buttons here but deep underlying muscles. Remember, as your muscles become tighter, they start strangling you...squeezing your arteries and closing off your circulation.

Massaging Across Muscles

Press in with the fingers, feeling for hard, tight muscles lying along the bone of the arm. Use the tips of the fingers and also the thumb when necessary.

Important: Massage *across* these muscles (from side to side), not with them as you do in reflex massage. Massage all the way up the arm, working the fingers on all sides of the arm and pressing in as you massage. If you find muscles that feel like steel bands, spend more time on these, but do not overdo it at first.

After you have massaged all the way up the arm, massage the muscles in the neck. See Photo 39. If you find these to be tight, spend some time massaging them to loosen them up. This also will help prevent a stroke by freeing the circulation of fresh blood to the brain. After you get these muscles loosened up, go to the muscles in the chest, especially on the left side. Massage *across* all the muscles in this area starting from the arm, under the arm and shoulder on down across the chest. Work on any muscles that might feel tight to your fingers. If any of these muscles are too tight to loosen with the fingers, use a vinegar pack to help loosen them and increase the circulation.

If it is hard for you to do this deep massage, another person might do it for you with better results. Just remember that tight muscles can cause a heart attack, so along with the methods of aiding your heart with reflex massage and diet, be sure that you keep these muscles to the heart loose and pliable.

Now let me give you a few hints on diet for your heart.

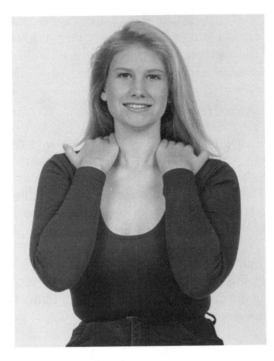

Photo 39: Position for massaging reflexes in the neck and shoulders.

How Reflexology and Diet Help the Heart and Prevent Strokes

The Importance of Vitamin E

Wilfred E. Shute, M.D., tells us in his book, *Vitamin E for Ailing and Healthy Hearts,* that coronary thrombosis, the major cause of heart attack death, is the greatest single killer in the world today. You may be surprised to know that coronary thrombosis was unknown as a disease entity in 1900 and apparently hardly existed at that time.

The late Dr. Paul Dudley White wrote: "When I graduated from medical school in 1911, I had never heard of coronary thrombosis, which is one of the chief threats to life in the United States and Canada today." How do we explain why a disease entity that did not occur prior to 1910 has become a greater ravager of human life than any plague recorded in history?

Historical Cause of Thrombosis Heart Attacks

When new and more efficient milling methods were introduced into the manufacture of wheat flour, permitting for the first time the complete stripping away of the highly perishable wheat germ, the diet of western man lost one of its best sources of vitamin E. Flour milling underwent this great change around the turn of the century, and it became widespread in 1910. For your heart's sake, take vitamin E every day and press heart reflexes as in Photo 5.

Dr. Shute tells us, "Vitamin E is, in addition to its other properties, a superb antithrombin in the bloodstream." Not only will vitamin E dissolve clots, but circulating in the blood of a healthy individual it will prevent thrombi (clots) from forming.

How Vitamin B-6 Prevents Heart Attacks and Strokes

According to research at Harvard University and Massachusetts Institute of Technology (MIT), vitamin B-6 can prevent heart attacks and strokes. Many doctors now claim that cholesterol is not the cause of heart disease and strokes. Experts believe that the real culprit is an amino acid called homocysteine and that vitamin B-6 eliminates the harmful substance from the body. Drs. Stephen A. Raymond and Edward R. Gruberg, MIT scientists, have concluded after two years of research that homocysteine, a by-product of high-protein diets, is the real cause of hardening of the arteries, which in turn causes heart attacks and strokes.

The Power of an Unusual Vitamin

Drs. Gruberg and Raymond are neurophysiologists—researchers specializing in the study of the nervous system. To get sufficient vitamin B-6, they say, you should either take B-6 supplements or eat more fruits, vegetables, whole grains, and nuts. At the same time, you should cut down on meat, eggs, and dairy products. When these high-protein foods are digested, the amino acid homocysteine is produced in the blood. Dr. Raymond tells us that homocysteine can harden and narrow the arteries by somehow stimulating the growth of cells along the delicate inner arterial walls.

Vitamin B-6 prevents the accumulation of homocysteine in the blood, thus dramatically reducing the risk of hardening of the arteries, which is the main cause of heart attack and stroke. Studies have shown that people with heart disease tend to have a vitamin B-6 deficiency and to have homocysteine acid in their blood. These doctors believe the Food and Drug Administration's recommended daily allowance of 2 milligrams of B-6 is far too low. They tell us that they supplement their own diets with 25 to 50 milligrams of B-6 daily. If these doctors who have made scientific studies of the importance of vitamin B-6 use it in their own diets, we had better take a hint from the experts and do likewise.

Heart Attacks and Strokes Prevented with a Vitamin

There is a growing belief among doctors that vitamin C can prevent heart attacks and strokes. The studies—one at the Medical University of South Carolina and two at Louisiana State University Medical Center—revealed that vitamin C reduces the tendency of blood platelets to stick together and cause clots.

Researchers note that this tendency, which is called "platelet aggregation," contributes to heart attacks and strokes. In the South Carolina study, Dr. Kay Sarji and fellow researchers gave eight healthy volunteers two grams of vitamin C daily for seven days. Blood was drawn before and after the test. Clotting agents were mixed with the blood, and the clotting of the blood was measured. In most cases platelet aggregation was reduced by more than 50 percent.

Miracles by Another Vitamin

Studies in Russia have proven that B-15 improves heartbeats in patients with heart disease. Dr. Richard Passwater tells us, "They have also shown that vitamin B-15 quickens the healing of scar tissue and limits the side effects of heart drugs when used with it."

The most recent studies have shown that B-15 is also effective in the liver for transporting fats.

It makes blood levels of cholesterol, some other fats, and certain hormones normal again. This regulating effect is unusual because if the levels are too low, it will bring them up; if they are too high, it will lower them. B-15 also has antiaging effects, keeping the cells alive and healthy by supplying proper amounts of oxygen to them. The recommended dosage is 150 milligrams per day.

I hope that this will encourage you to take these special vitamins to protect your heart. Of course, other substances, such as the other B complex vitamins and potassium, are also important to a healthy heart.

Healthy Circulatory System Reduces Risk of Heart Attack and Strokes

Prevention is the best known factor to reduce chances of a stroke, which is a devastating experience and can cause frightening damage. Prevent the risk of heart attack or stroke by keeping blood pressure down. Eat less fat and fewer cholesterol-rich foods and decrease your intake of sodium.

Better circulation will help ward off potentially harming heart problems and will help create the natural free flow of life surging through the body, for a natural balance and healthy harmony. Give a complete reflex workout, and concentrate on the circulatory system for a renewal of sparkling health!

One man wrote us with this wonderful news:

Husband Stopped Wife's Black-out Spells with Reflexology

Dear Mrs. Carter,

My wife has had black-out spells for the last thirty years. She once fell during a black-out and broke her leg. I couldn't understand why all the doctors and specialists we were referred to for this problem couldn't find what was wrong and do something for her. We had no success at all; they just prescribed pills that didn't work.

I started over a year ago giving my wife reflexology treatments, and she hasn't had any black-out spells since. I feel as though, with your help, I have accomplished a great deal. My wife recently went to Europe on a trip for a month, and she had no problems at all. I feel as though I made a breakthrough on her case with reflexology. I am very proud of myself, and happy for her. I just can't believe I did this and all those doctors and specialists had no success at all.

Thank you.

—Mr. J.W. Florida

Wife Tells How Reflexology Saves Husband from Stroke

Dear Mrs. Carter,

Ten years ago last June my husband had a major stroke and I believe that if I had known then what I know now I could have saved him much suffering and disability. He has made a wonderful recovery with the help of good doctors and loving care. He had carotid artery surgery which was successful but for six months he could not speak, and for weeks his right side was paralyzed but no one worked harder than he to get well. I was fortunate to have a friend who was a speech therapist and she loaned me some of her books and I worked with my husband until he was able to talk again. He can't always say just what he wants to and he can't always think of people's names, but we don't grieve over what he has lost; we are most thankful for what he still has and can do.

The night before Easter, my husband took his bath and then came into the living room where I was crocheting and he was shaking his hands as if they had gone to sleep. I looked up at him and saw he was trying to talk. He moved his lips but no sound came out. I told him to sit in the lounge chair and I started working on his feet. His condition really frightened me because this was exactly the same way his massive stroke had started ten years before. I worked his diaphram and solar plexus, his adrenals, and his brain. Then I worked the whole foot but concentrated on the first three areas mentioned. In about fifteen minutes he was able to speak and there were no visible signs of damage. I work on his feet almost every day, and he works on his hands several times per day and really enjoys his "little ball with the knobs on it." My husband is seventy-six years old and cares for five dairy goats. He has a little shop where he repairs lawn mowers and other air-cooled motors, We have a garden and can most of our food. I am a YOUNG seventy-five years old, and work full time as a dental assistant and I love it!!! I expect to be an active reflexologist for many years.

Sincerely yours,

—L.N.

NATURE'S STIMULATOR

Above all, remember that walking is nature's perfect body stimulator. It increases the oxygen flow to the lungs, which sends rich blood to every part of your body. It feeds every cell from your brain to your toes, and it makes your heart work. When your heart has to work, it will get stronger every day. Of course, you will do this under a doctor's care if you have a history of heart problems. Doctors are telling patients to get out and walk, run, or jog. Walk briskly, swinging the arms in rhythm, the left arm and the right leg, then the right arm and the left leg. All the vitamins in the world will not give you a strong heart without *exercise!*

REFLEXOLOGY IN CASES OF EMERGENCY

I wish that everyone would learn the few simple methods for treating heart attacks with reflex massage. It is so easy to do. Anyone, from an aged person to a very young child, can safely use the technique of reflexology when there is a sudden emergency and they are not able to use any other method to aid the victim until help arrives. Knowing how to massage the reflexes correctly might even save your own life. I have prevented several heart attacks, as have many of my students; thus, patients have been saved from a badly damaged heart, or death, while waiting for the paramedics and the attention of a doctor. I am sure that many lives would be saved and that the recovery rate would be much higher if everyone knew a few simple techniques of reflex massage, especially sports enthusiasts and people who like the great outdoors.

Every year we are saddened by the high rate of deaths from heart attacks during the hunting season. People start out with such a happy anticipation of adventure away from all the confusion and pressure of city life. (Most of the people are in poor physical condition.) They overindulge in alcohol, they overexert bodies that are not used to strenuous exercise, and disaster strikes. Their hearts give out and many of them never see their families again. *Don't let this happen to you!*

Check the reflex buttons to your heart to make sure that it is in good condition. Use reflex massage to strengthen and build up your heart *before* you put it to strenuous unaccustomed pressure. I will tell you how to do this later in this chapter, but right now I would like you to learn to use these special methods of reflexology on yourself and also on others in case you are ever faced with an emergency heart attack. Remember that the following methods are *by no means a substitute for proper medical care* but are to be used in an emergency when no help is available. They may be used in conjunction with standard medical care.

If You Have Symptoms of Heart Malfunction

Let us say you are up in the mountains and you suddenly begin to feel out of breath with pains in the chest or other symptoms of heart malfunction. Because you know how to use reflex massage, *you will not panic.* You will sit down immediately. If you are too weak to dig into the reflexes in your left hand, squeeze the little finger of your left hand. See Photo 40. Hold it tightly. This should relax you enough to enable you to dig in the palm of the left hand and hunt for a sore spot. Also massage the area below the little finger. Do not let the pain of the reflex button stop you. Use whatever method is easier for you. See Photo 28. Relax! Tension causes a strain on the heart. You may have to press quite hard on the hand reflexes, or you might even use a stick, but get into those reflexes and massage hard. Massage the sore button first, then work all around it, then go back to it until the soreness eases up. If you get a twinge of pain in the left shoulder, stick your thumb into that spot and massage for a few seconds or hold a steady pressure on it, then return to massaging the reflexes in the left hand. When you feel better, you might take off your left shoe and massage the reflexes on the little toe and the pad below it. Remember that the heart is a large organ and takes up quite a large space in your

chest. Since you do not know which part of the heart is malfunctioning, it is good to massage the whole area after you have massaged out
most of the painful reflex buttons.

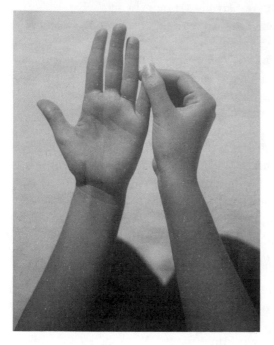

Photo 40: Pinching the little finger on the left hand to
help a malfunctioning heart.
(Pinching the little toe on
the left foot will be equally
beneficial.)

Helping Someone Else

If a person having difficulty is unable to perform reflexology on his or
her own hands, I suggest that you take off his shoes and on the left
foot massage the little toe and the pad below the little toe. See
Diagram 5. This will probably be quite painful, but massage the
whole area. As soon as you feel that you have him stabilized, go to the
center of the pad in the big toe and press in hard. If it is too sore, use
a lighter pressure. This can be very painful for some people. This is
the reflex to the pituitary gland, which will help send a flow of life
energy throughout the endocrine glands. You can easily use all these
methods of reflexology on yourself if you find it necessary.

If someone else shows signs that might indicate a heart attack, you can also use the same procedure as I have told you to use on yourself. Also, to improve a failing heartbeat, use the flat section of your fist to bang on the part of the body where the head joins the neck. See Diagram 6B. This stimulates a nerve that speeds up the heartbeat.

Since we are talking of emergency treatment where there is no help available, I give you Dr. Lavitan's method of treating a severe heart attack.

Reflexology Saves a Life

Dr. Lavitan tells us of a patient who had a heart attack right in his waiting room. It happened so quickly that by the time the doctor reached his side the victim had no pulse or blood pressure and had begun to shake all over. Death must have been seconds away. The doctor had nothing to lose, so he grabbed the man's left hand and began to really dig in and massage the palm. See Photo 28. At first, there was no reaction. Then the victim began to gasp for air. The pulse finally started up, stopped, started again, fluttered, and finally began to get into rhythm. In this case, an ambulance came and the man recovered nicely.

Another doctor's testimonial is of a woman who suffered from severe angina pains, which occurred at least once a month. They were so agonizing and came on so suddenly that she always lived in fear of the next attack. She was on regular medication, including nitroglycerin, yet her medication didn't really stop the attacks or eliminate the pain. When the doctor examined her, he spent ten minutes massaging these reflexes that I have just explained to you. This happened a year and a half ago, and she hasn't had a single attack since the first treatment.

Vacation Saved by Reflexology

I was on vacation with a friend much younger than I. We had rented a motel room on the second floor, and as we were unloading the car she grabbed a suitcase and took off up the stairs. When I got to the top I noticed her sitting on the suitcase. She was acting very strangely and was pale and sweating. She said she was dizzy, couldn't see well, was too weak to get up. I grabbed her left hand and had her hold pressure on her little finger while I pressed some of the body reflexes to the heart. I also worked on the reflexes on her head. After a few minutes she felt better and walked into the room. Because we were in a strange town, she refused to see a doctor. I made her stay in bed the next day while I worked on the reflexes to the heart and also to the endocrine glands. We only missed one day of our vacation, and when she got home her doctor said she was okay. She was a school teacher and not used to much exercise. Overstraining the heart can be dangerous; knowing reflexology could save a life.

I am sure that you will agree with me that reflexology is something that everyone should learn. I hope that you never have to use this emergency information, but if you need it just once in your life, you will be glad that you knew what to do.

Relief of Heart Pains and Headaches

Dear Mildred Carter,

A church group of forty-, fifty-, and sixty-year-olds was climbing a very steep hill; we were zig-zagging our way up. Part of the way up and then again at the top, a man and woman were short of breath and were having chest pains with racing hearts. I massaged the heart reflex on the lady's left hand and told her how to do it. Then I massaged the man's heart reflex. Both experienced immediate relief and couldn't thank me enough.

On three other occasions, headaches disappeared almost as fast. Thank you so much.

—Mrs. D.W., Registered Nurse

REFLEXOLOGY TEST FOR POSSIBLE HEART PROBLEMS

Now let me tell you of a few simple techniques to use to make sure that your heart is in perfect condition. You should take this test a few weeks before you plan to do things that will put an extra strain on your heart—things that you are not accustomed to doing every day such as sports, hiking, shoveling snow in the winter, and so on.

Earlier in this chapter, I told you of several methods of checking the reflexes for the heart. Here is another method as described by Dr. Lavitan.

Press hard on the top section of the left thumb pad. If you don't have much strength in your hands, you might use the hand massager, which is described in Chapter 36 in this book. See Photo 28. (It is wise always to have in your possession a magic reflex massager, a hand massager, a reflex comb, and a tongue probe.)

This method of reflexology can warn you of an oncoming heart attack. According to Dr. Lavitan, when you dig into the top part of the thumb pad and it hurts, it is telling you that the blood vessels going to your heart are constricting, cutting off the blood supply and reducing its oxygen. If the bottom half of the pad is where it is tender or sore, then the arteries in your heart are getting "clogged up."

If it is just a little bit sore, the possibility of a heart attack may exist but is more remote. If you should go "ouch, that really hurts" and you have to stop because it is so painful, the chances are greater that a heart attack might occur. It is much better to be forewarned of danger of a heart attack, so that you can do something to strengthen the heart immediately. Check with your chiropractor or a physician. There are many other things that could be wrong, but you have been given the warning in time to prevent an attack if you are in danger of one.

Important note: If the thumb on the right hand is also sore on these pads, you are probably not in danger of a heart attack. It is probably telling you a different story.

Dr. Lavitan says, "I particularly like this heart attack test because it's quick. It doesn't cost anything, you don't need any equipment, and you can do it yourself in fifteen seconds."

In some cases, a person will have a "diagnosed" heart condition—usually angina—and yet the left palm will not be painful. This is because many cases of angina may not be a true heart condition but simply a misplaced rib. The misplaced rib may cause muscle spasms that feel like heart pain or a heart attack. If you suspect that this might be true in your situation or that of a friend, check with a good chiropractor. (According to Dr. Lavitan, this viewpoint is shared by the eminent cardiologist Dr. Wilfred Shute.)

The Doctor Had Given Up Hope

Dear Mrs. Carter,

My seventy-three-year-old sister took the swine flu shot. After a few days, she was taken to the hospital with a heart condition. The doctor called it heart failure. When he had given her a matter of hours to live, my other sister called me. I lived in another town thirty miles away. I called a cab and rushed to the hospital. I found her with little pulse—her heart was very weak. I gave her the reflexology heart treatment, and in less than fifteen minutes, her pulse was back to normal. She was noticing people in her room and was able to hold a conversation with me. This was on a Saturday night, and about 8:30 a.m. on Tuesday morning, her doctor released her to go home. He did not know what had made her well so quickly. Should I have told him?

—M.O.

Reflexology Helps Calm Heart

Dear Mrs. Carter,

I am a woman, sixty-two years old, and I have been in the medical field for a number of years. I just got over two operations for cancer and chemotherapy this past year plus I have high blood pressure. I've been under a great deal of stress and have been working very hard in the garden and yard for long hours. Recently I had an irregular heartbeat for a day and a half. I did not call the doctor, but instead I soaked my feet and massaged the reflex area under my toe and got up and walked around. I was surprised and delighted to find my pulse was regular again. What a relief—after an afternoon, night and morning worrying but trying not to panic. It wasn't psychosomatic, as I have had pounding of the heart other times through the years upon heavy exertion and knew this time I had just worked too hard and too long.

Thanking you. Very truly yours,

—E.G.

Reflexology Brings Down Blood Pressure

Dear Mrs. Carter,

God bless you for a good inexpensive way to stay healthy. I am seventy-four years young. I am taking B.P. pills and my cholesterol is 246, my blood pressure is under control, but I can't seem to get the cholesterol down. I am walking three miles a day with three friends, it takes us one hour. I use reflexology on my body all the time to stay healthy.

Thank you. Love and Prayers,

—H.P.

Reflexology May Have Saved Life

Dear Mrs. Carter,

During the past week I have had some rather stressful experiences. Someone had broken into my home and walked off with some irreplaceable valuables. Then, along with that I have had other trying experiences. Seemed as though it would never end. Usually, I am able to handle rough times and come out serene. Very frequently, too, I've been able to help others regain their peace and calm, but for some reason last week I felt a dire need of help. Although I prayed, the burden still lagged on, one trial after the other. I felt as though it was making me sick. I got up at 3:30 this morning—I picked up your reflexology book and started massaging the reflex to the heart. I massaged the pad of the little toe, in toward the center of the foot, nothing happened. I then moved up toward the little toe. Just beneath the little toe toward the fourth toe, I felt a sore spot and began to press it out. All of a sudden a sharp, shooting pain rushed all the way up my left leg, straight up the left side of my body to the heart. I bit tightly on my lips and continued to work it out. I felt as if it were a small bead that kept slipping beneath my finger as I pressed. My hand was a bit tired, but a small voice within me kept on saying, "Be not weary in well doing." So I kept on working it out until the pain stopped. I worked over the whole area of reflex to the heart. In fact, I massaged both feet and went back to sleep.

Thank you...You may have saved my life!!!

God Bless You.

—A.B. New York

Blood Transfusions Stopped After Use of Reflexology

Dear Mrs. Carter,

I have a friend who had to have blood transfusions because of aplastic anemia and a bone marrow test. She was in very bad shape. The spleen has been the most effective reflex in helping this woman. I used the technique of warming her feet (with a hair dryer), then wrapping them, for she had very cold feet. Your method of rubbing hands together for friction and then applying them helped her so much, for her feet were sore to a gentle touch. This worked wonders. Her blood and bone marrow have improved and now she no longer needs blood transfusions. She was sent to North Carolina to new doctors and showed improvement from an 8.1 blood count to 9.6. We are very happy with her improvement. She also gained *two* much needed pounds. Reflexology is GREAT!!!

—Mrs. S.C.

Reflexology Keeps Me Healthy

Dear Mrs. Carter,

In early childhood I had a bout with whooping cough and the three-day measles. All the rest of my life has been free of contagious diseases...even though I have visited the sick. Since this is also true of my family, I can only assume that a good, strong thymus is part of our heritage. Every relative I ever had, passed on from heart disease or attack. Nothing else!! So that's why I sometimes get a pinpoint twinge at the foot heart reflex, when in bed or sitting in a chair. So now I'm digging at it when the signal comes. My insurance company's doctor can't find anything wrong but Mother Nature is talking to me.

Love, V.M.

HOW REFLEXOLOGY HELPS GET RID OF VARICOSE VEINS

Varicose veins appear when there is interference in the circulatory system. Often the inadequate functioning of blood can cause a dull ache or tired feeling in the legs accompanied by blue lines.

A neighbor of my daughter asked if I knew of any way to dissolve the blue lines in her legs. She had been suffering with this problem for about four months. Ronda works in an office where she sits in one place for several hours a day. Unfortunately, her inactivity worsens the impaired circulation. She is a tall girl, and said that she crosses her legs most of the time, which also adds to her problem.

I suggested that she work the reflexes on her feet and hands, and gave her some exercises to increase circulation. First I explained the wonderful advantage of working on the hands. They are so convenient, and one can work the reflexes while at their desk, or anywhere, and at anytime. One very basic technique is to place your thumb in the palm of one hand and wrap your fingers around the back. Use your thumb to press into the reflexes on the palm side. This will feel as though you are trying to pinch your thumb and fingers together, right through your hand. Move your thumb in slow, small pressing circles. Work the thumb, and each finger, giving special attention to every joint, and the webs between all fingers. Work back and forth across your whole hand, to the wrist.

Now work the wrist and up your forearm, as this is the "referral area" to your calves, and will benefit circulation to your legs and feet. Repeat on other hand, wrist and arm. See Photo "B" on page 104. (Use this referral technique in advanced cases, when ankles are swollen or leg cramps occur.)

Increase Your Circulation

I suggest you use the foot roller to increase circulation and get your blood moving. This will stimulate many reflexes on the bottom of your feet, and at the same time, you will be moving your legs and encouraging the blood to move throughout your whole body. See Photos 42 and 43 in Chapter 13.

Activity is important; walking and swimming are wonderful exercises, to improve venous blood flow. Even when the weather is bad, you can take a brisk walk around the house or workplace. Walking up and down the stairs for ten minutes, four or five times every day will help keep blood moving and legs healthy. Take the opportunity to walk barefoot whenever you can, as this exercises your foot muscles and improves circulation. When in motion, your calves will start contracting and pushing blood upward. However, when you must sit or stand still for hours at a time, you lose the benefit of this pumping action.

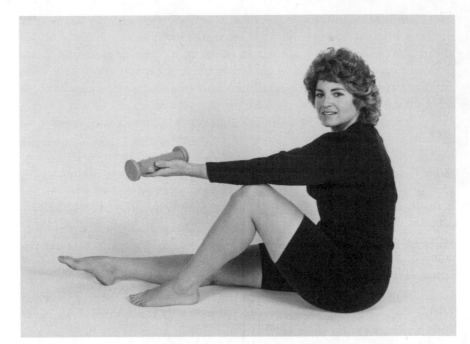

Referral Areas are: Hand/Foot, Forearm/Calf, Upper Arm/Thigh,
Wrist/Ankle, and Knee/Elbow

Photo "B": Working the REFERRAL AREA to the corresponding energy
zone will enhance recovery of a swollen or sensitive area.

Example: Speed recovery to hurt or inflamed foot by working the "referral
area" . . . (on hand), on the same side of the body.

Remember, varicose veins have a tendency to get worse if adequate preventive measures are not taken, so stand up and move
around, raise and lower yourself on the balls and toes of your feet,
then on the heels and sides of your feet...rotate your feet, make wide
circles in one direction and then in the other..."pump" your feet by
pointing your toes toward your face, then away from you. Repeat
about sixty times once every hour. These exercises are so simple and
will only take a few minutes of your time, yet they will add circulation
and speed the healing forces within your legs.

Elevate Your Feet

Often symptoms of heaviness and fatigue accompany varicose veins. When you elevate your feet about six inches above your heart, it reduces the pressure in the veins and reverses the gravitational pull. So make sure you elevate both feet whenever possible. A slant board will help move pools of blood that may have accumulated in the veins, back to your heart.

Why Increased Fiber in Your Diet Is Important

A high-fiber diet is very important to your system because without adequate roughage, the system may become constipated. When this happens, the natural urge is to strain, but strain to excrete hard stools puts extra stress on the veins in your legs, making it hard for them to return blood up to your heart.

Being overweight can also cause additional varicose vein problems because excess pressure on the legs contributes to the inability of muscles to push blood upward.

Remember to eat living foods such as vegetables and fruit, especially those rich in minerals that will help relieve constipation and aid your body's circulatory system. These are the foods from the root crops such as onions, garlic, carrots, and radishes.

Studies have shown that vitamin E supplements of 400 I.U. and 50 mg of zinc daily will help open collateral circulation in the legs. Remember what Dr. Shute tells us about Vitamin E. See page 90. Vitamin E cream can be applied directly onto the skin, which will help if your legs are dry or feel achy and tired.

Ronda reported that by elevating her feet, using the foot and ankle rotation exercise, eating better foods, and taking vitamin E and zinc, she has noticed great improvements. She feels that the reflex foot roller has helped her circulation and claims the veins are less inflated from the pressure of blood, her legs now look and feel better.

You too can produce healthy results by using these healing methods to enable damaged valves within the veins to send trapped blood back to your heart. Soon you will be moving freely and feel a new zest for life.

CHAPTER 10

How Reflexology Helps the Stomach and Digestion

Many things can cause an upset stomach and poor digestion. Look at Diagram 9, and you will see how several factors can contribute to your discomfort. After the food goes into the stomach, it is affected by the liver and the gallbladder and then the pancreas as it passes through the small intestines into the large intestine (colon) before it is expelled as waste.

REFLEXES TO THE STOMACH

See Diagrams 7 and 8. Notice the location of the reflex buttons to the stomach, the liver, and the gallbladder. Take the middle finger and press into the reflex button marked stomach. Is it sore? Move the finger up or down a little to find the area that is painful. See Photo 4. Usually, the stomach reflexes are quite sensitive to a little pressure. Move the finger to the right and press on the reflex buttons to the liver and the gallbladder. Then move the finger down to the small intestine reflex. Now, move the finger over and up to the colon reflexes and press here along the waistline and on several buttons on both sides of the abdomen as shown in the charts. After you have located these reflex buttons, you may use three fingers to press and hold, use the fingers on both hands simultaneously, or use the reflex roller. See Photo 7.

I have already told you how to activate these reflexes in a previous chapter, but I will repeat it here. Press and hold for the count of three, and then release for the count of three and repeat. Do this three times to each reflex. If you are having digestion problems, you must also use this same technique on the navel reflex. See Photo 3.

There are other less important reflexes to the stomach and other parts of the body, but to keep this simple and easy to follow I am giving you the more important ones to work on. Remember, the stomach can also be the cause of headaches.

Before I knew about reflexology, one evening my husband had a bad case of indigestion. He took every kind of antacid remedy that we had in the house with no relief. Finally, I suggested he take a little vinegar in water. He did this and got immediate relief.

RELIEF FROM ULCERS WITH REFLEXOLOGY

There have been many cases of ulcers relieved by reflexology. One of the main reasons is the almost immediate release from built-up nervous tension that usually is the main cause of the ulcer. The reflexes in the feet are usually the most relaxing. Just use the reflex massage method as taught earlier in this book. Next come the reflexes on the hands—search for "ouch" spots all over the hands and the feet, and when you find them, massage them for several seconds.

In all these reflex areas, you may find it easier if you use the reflex devices described elsewhere in this book. I am speaking of the foot roller, the hand probe, and the magic massager. Also, the reflex roller is indispensable for searching out and massaging the reflexes on all parts of the body. The tongue probe is especially good for all types of stomach problems. See Photo 22.

Anyone with an ulcer or a long history of stomach problems should be under the care of a good naturopathic doctor, chiropractor, or medical doctor.

Remember, first you must get rid of stress. It is well known that a dog will not keep an ulcer if left on his own. He merely goes and lies down and relaxes and the ulcer vanishes. Can you do this? With the help of reflexology, you can!

Quiet your nerves with love for your fellow man. Anger and upset is poison in your bloodstream that goes to every cell in your body, so strive to relax. Massage the reflexes to the endocrine glands and especially the pituitary gland.

I highly recommend that you take Propolis to help cure an ulcer. Propolis is another one of nature's cures; derived from bees, it has an uncanny healing property.

Ulcers Went Away

Dear Mrs. Carter,

A few years ago, I had ulcers in my stomach. After using reflexology I felt much better and my ulcers went away. I now have a very good appetite for food and have gained a few needed pounds. Also, my lungs are much clearer when I use the reflexology methods.

—S.S.

HOW REFLEXOLOGY HELPS RELIEVE FLATULENCE, CONSTIPATION, DIARRHEA, NAUSEA AND INDIGESTION

How to Eliminate Excessive Gas

Many people may be bothered with flatulence, or a buildup of gases that cause distention, and often a great deal of discomfort. You will be amazed at how reflexology helps alleviate these problems. You must remember how important your diet is too.

Work the reflexes to the digestive system (liver, stomach, intestines, gallbladder, and pancreas) where foods are broken down into tiny pieces. Also work the reflexes to the colon and duodenum to release excessive gas buildup in the stomach or intestines. Pressing your fingers into a painful area in the stomach usually moves the gas bubble so you no longer suffer the discomfort.

Exercise for Constipation and Release of Flatulence

Exercise is a great way to get waste matter moving through the body. Stimulation brings needed blood and oxygen to the intestines that helps them to work properly. It is very beneficial to bend at the mid-section to loosen up stools. This knee-to-chest exercise moves the digestive system and relaxes the back. Lie on your back and bring both knees up. Clasp your hands underneath both folded knees, then rock gently back and forth.

You may find that bending one knee at a time is best for you. Breathe deeply, and repeat four or five times; then change legs. Sit with your back straight when using a toilet facility, to make sure your colon is not pinched.

How to Use Reflexology to Help Stomach Troubles

Hold your left palm in front of you. With the thumb of your right hand, work the soft spongy area found near the pad of the thumb and near the web. Work this area with a rolling, pressing motion for a few minutes. If you feel nauseated, do not continue pressure on that hand. Try working the same area on the right hand. The stomach lies mostly on the left side, but is affected by the same reflexes in each hand. See Photo "C."

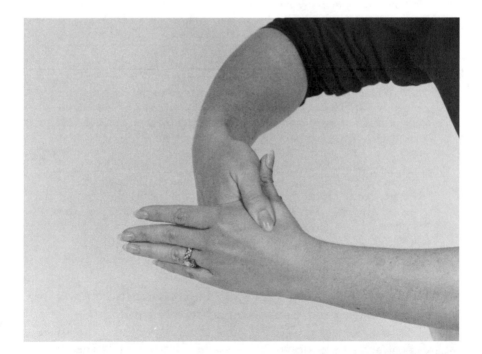

Photo "C": Pressure point to relieve pain in many parts of the body, including abdominal pain, headaches and cramps.

If your thyroid is not functioning properly, your whole system may be sluggish. A low thyroid function can cause bowel contractions to slow down, therefore slowing the movement of wastes out of your body. Use reflexology to work the reflexes of the thyroid gland to speed up its function.

Constipation can be a problem for those who do not get enough physical activity.

> Nolla, a lady in her late seventies, was bedridden following an accident. She failed to heed the urge to defecate, as it was too painful for her to get in and out of bed, and this caused her to suffer with constipation. Her feces remained too long in the colon and became dry and hard, and difficult to eliminate. Things became worse for her as she developed hemorrhoids.
>
> Nolla needed increased circulation throughout her body, as her glands and organs were becoming dormant. She needed to renew her health and vitality. So I gave her a magic massager to use for two minutes on one hand, then she was to change the massager to the other hand, using it again for two minutes. She was to use it only twice the first day, once in the morning and once in the evening. This little massager is very powerful in stimulating the reflexes to many glands at once. Two days later I checked on her and she told me she felt the stimulation of life and vitality surging through her whole body.
>
> Reflexology treatments and the use of her magic reflex massager helped her get back on the road to recovery.
>
> We know how important muscular activity is to the digestive tract, so we gave Nolla a few reflexology lessons. She learned how to work the reflexes in her hands by holding the magic reflex massager and combing over the reflexes by pressing the teeth of a comb into the center of her hand.
>
> We also changed her diet from refined foods to one with fruits, steamed vegetables, grain cereals, bran, and sauerkraut. Soon she had relief from constipation.
>
> Reflexology and a change in diet gave her complete relief from constipation.

Diarrhea Helped with Use of Reflexology

Elimination problems can mean the difference between working, vacationing, playing sports, or staying close to a bathroom.

The large intestine (colon) is meant to absorb liquid from solid wastes that are passed down to the small intestine. Diarrhea results when there is interference in that absorption, which will cause the bowel to secrete, not absorb, liquid. Or when the passage of wastes go through the bowel so fast that there is insufficient time for any fluid to be absorbed. You will want to work the reflex to the heart to bring about a normal rhythm, to prevent low blood pressure. Work the kidney reflex to balance the elimination of fluid and waste.

There are numerous reasons for extreme looseness of bowel movements; we won't go into all the different causes. If this is a problem for you, it can be painful, inconvenient, and very frustrating. If you're going on vacation, especially to underdeveloped countries with poor sanitation, drink only bottled water and juices. Remember to use the bottled water when brushing your teeth, and don't use ice in your drinks. Make sure the refrigeration is good before eating fish, mayonnaise, or meats, and avoid fruits, unless you peel them yourself.

To help stop diarrhea, you will want to strengthen your digestive system. Lay down on your back and place your middle finger two inches above your navel. Press and move in a small circular motion, not lifting your finger from the skin for about two minutes. Now move your finger down a bit in the direction of a clock, and press with a circular movement, moving all the way around your navel with this system. Then relax.

Work the thyroid reflex to regulate body functions. Your kidney, stomach, intestines, liver, and colon should all be stimulated with a good reflexology workout to relieve diarrhea and enjoy healthy regularity.

Diarrhea does not create inner cleansing as some people think. On the contrary, it may cause nutritional deficiency because as the nutrients are moved on through the body so fast, they cannot be absorbed. If diarrhea lasts too long, it may lead to malnutrition and will cause a loss of water and salts from the body.

Nutritional deficiency will affect your immune system and you may suffer premature aging. So do not let this happen to you. Use reflexology to normalize your system and try a change in your diet.

Diet Change Could Help

Pectin will act as a binding substance and tighten up (normalize) loose bowels. Foods such as bananas and apples contain pectin. Add them to your diet for beneficial results.

Stop diarrhea by fixing a bowl of two chopped bananas, one cup of plain yogurt and one tablespoon of bran. The fiber will normalize the functioning of the intestines, while the pectin in the bananas will fight against diarrhea and replenish your body with lost potassium, magnesium, and other nutrients that may have been drained out. Bran will help thicken those loose, liquid stools. This recipe should help firm up stools in two to three days.

Alleviate Nausea

Some friends of my son-in-law had gone on a fishing trip out in the Pacific Ocean. They left San Diego, California, early one morning, excited about the "big ones" they planned to pull in. Within two hours the fun was over. Rough waters and scrambled egg sandwiches had most of the guys hanging over the sides of the boat. The next day, they asked if there was any kind of reflex button that would alleviate nausea. The first reflex that came to mind was the point on the inside of the wrist, between the two large tendons. The button can be found about three fingers from the wrist. Press deeply for several minutes until the button starts to ache. This point takes a little longer to work for nausea. For severe nausea it may take twenty-five minutes or longer. See Photo 38.

I also told them that if this happens again to lie down and loosen any clothing that may be tight or uncomfortable. Breathing slow and deeply will help relax the stomach. I suggested the technique for relieving upset stomachs, which is pressing the stomach with the fingers of the left hand. See Photo 2.

They said they would have tried every method of self-care they could out there, because medicine would not stay down. They were happy with the tips on reflexology; however, they told me that their next fishing trip is going to be from shore.

Indigestion Cured with Reflexology

Dear Mrs. Carter,

Some time last year, after I had read your book, *Body Reflexology*, I developed a bad case of indigestion one evening which felt like a cramping pain just behind the navel. On the theory "if it hurts, hurt it back" I jammed my thumb deep into my navel for a minute or two...and got immediate relief, along with a satisfying belch of a lot of trapped gas! I get this kind of cramping sensation from stressful situations such as having to deal with a negative person or watching a graphic news story on TV that "turns my stomach." Now I can turn it right-side-up again!

I have certainly found your books useful. I have used them to help me stay away from doctors and surgeons for years...they're even better than apples!!!

Best wishes,

—L.M.D.

Hiccups Stopped with Reflexology

When I was in Hawaii, one evening I walked into a store for something. The clerk was getting ready to close when an agitated young woman and her husband came in. She asked for an alkalizer or something similar to stop her terrible hiccups.

I told her husband to press, "Here," pointing to my stomach. He looked puzzled but walked over and pressed *my* stomach, much to my surprise! I said, "No! No! Do it to her—like this." Standing in back of her, I reached around her and pressed into her stomach with the fingers of both my hands, about halfway between the breastbone and the navel, holding about three seconds. She looked at me in pleasant surprise and said, "They're gone, the hiccups are all gone!" Her husband asked, "Are you a doctor?"

The store clerk couldn't believe what she had witnessed.

Reflexology is just one of nature's greatest, yet simplest, methods of natural healing.

Addicted to Reflexology

Dear Mrs. Carter,

When I was about twenty-four years of age I had five hard spots rubbed out of my intestines by a masseur friend. Since that time (I am now eighty-five years old) I have used the practice on my stomach and intestines to relieve constipation and aches and pains caused by injuries. I am addicted to reflexology for myself, and also for my wife. Thank you for bringing your knowledge of body reflexology into our lives. All of your instructions are so simple and easy to follow. I am trying to register all of your instructions in my mind so I can use them on my wife and others who need natural healing.

—H.E.P.

CHAPTER 11

Diet, Vitamins, and Reflexology

When I was first introduced to reflexology, I was told not to recommend any other type of healing, as this would confuse people and they would not give credit to reflex massage when they recovered from illnesses. Before studying reflexology, I studied nutrition for several years because of my husband's early heart attack, so I did recommend what I had learned about diet and nutrition. I did not follow my teacher's instruction in this matter, and I have never recommended reflexology as the *only* healing therapy.

Dr. Gaylord Hauser, the famous nutritionist, tells us that as a young boy he lay dying in a hospital in Chicago. He had undergone many operations and injections for a tubercular hip that refused to heal. Finally, the doctors told his parents to take him home as there was nothing more they could do for him. He was sent home to die in the serenity of the Swiss mountains. There, an old man came to visit and told him that only living foods can make a living body. This man knew nothing about vitamins, proteins, minerals, and other nutrients, but the boy listened and followed the old man's advice by eating enormous amounts of fresh living foods (raw vegetables and fruit). They saved his life, and I believe that Dr. Hauser, in his nineties, is still enjoying good health in his Swiss mountains.

BREWER'S YEAST: WONDER FOOD

Dr. Hauser recommends brewer's yeast, which contains seventeen different vitamins, including all the B family; sixteen amino acids; and fourteen minerals, including the "trace" minerals held to be essential. It also contains 36 percent protein (sirloin steak may contain as little as 23 percent protein). Steak contains 22 percent fat, but brewer's yeast only contains 1 percent fat. We are talking about one tablespoon—eight grams—only 22 calories.

There are several different varieties now on the market that you may buy at your health food store. Do not confuse this for the yeast that is used in baking. Never eat fresh yeast that is made for baking!

THE VALUE OF BLACKSTRAP MOLASSES

My next favorite wonder food, recommended by Dr. Hauser, is unsulphured molasses or blackstrap molasses. It has some wonderful healing properties, not only when taken as a food but also when applied to cuts and abrasions.

Blackstrap molasses is very rich in iron and the B vitamins. Do *not* use the kind that is sold any place but at the health food stores. The kind sold elsewhere is made of mostly sugar, which you certainly do not want to use, unless you want to slowly poison your body and destroy your teeth.

Many people cannot tolerate the taste of blackstrap molasses, and I was one of those people. I tried every way to make it palatable because I knew of its high food value. I finally acquired a taste for it by using a very small amount at a time in warm or cold milk or water. Molasses is especially good for children and older people when taken at bedtime in place of a chocolate milk drink. You can get some added calcium by enriching your drink with powdered milk. We all need as much calcium as we can get.

I have also used blackstrap molasses as an enema for trouble in the colon and as a douche when there was any indication of trouble in that area. It has uncanny healing properties when it is used either internally or externally. It may also be held in the mouth to help alleviate a toothache or sores in the mouth.

Many times when I am overworked and feel washed out, a glass of blackstrap molasses and milk gives me a quick pickup when I don't have time for my reflexology pickup massage. To keep healthy the body needs every type of help that we can give it in these days of poisoned air, polluted and poisoned water, and questionable additives that replace the natural nutrients in our foods.

WHEAT GERM, A WONDER FOOD

Wheat germ is claimed to be worth its weight in gold. It is an outstanding source of vitamins B-1, B-2, B-6, and niacin. One-half cup provides a generous daily allowance of this important vitamin. It is rich in protein and provides nearly three times as much iron as other sources.

Fresh wheat germ is delicious sprinkled over hot or cold cereals. It also adds to the flavor and nutrition of any baked product such as biscuits, bread, cakes, and so on, and adds a nutty flavor to fresh fruits and salads.

Wheat germ is also a good source of vitamin E, which helps in healing many types of heart problems. So don't neglect to find ways to include wheat germ when preparing meals for your family. Along with reflex massage, this is another health bonus to help you stay young and live a long healthy life. Use raw wheat germ when it is available, and keep it stored in the refrigerator to retain its freshness.

THE WONDER OF YOGURT

Yogurt is credited for the longevity of the Bulgarians and natives of other countries who retain vigor, vitality, and youth to an extremely advanced age.

Yogurt is easily assimilated, it contains high-quality protein, and it supplies significant amounts of calcium and riboflavin (vitamin B-2) to the diet. It is an acceptable between-meal snack for a quick pickup and an excellent food to eat before going to bed. One cup of yogurt fortified with powdered skim milk gives you about 7 percent of the calories, 17 percent of the protein, 50 percent of the calcium, and 30 percent of the vitamin B-2 needed for a day's diet.

According to information from clinical tests, children who are fed yogurt grow much larger than do children who did not receive yogurt in their diet. If you want your children to grow into large adults, yogurt may be the answer. If your children are growing too fast, maybe you should not include yogurt in their diets and should give extra attention to the pituitary gland. See Chapter 8 on endocrine glands.

The Importance of Liquid Golden Oils for Sustained Energy and Smaller Waistlines

Fat seems to have a bad name these days, but we all need some fat. Fat is used as a source of sustained energy, as a heat insulation under the skin, and as a padding for the framework to round out the contours of the body.

Dr. Gaylord Hauser tells us that meals containing some fats have greater "staying power" because fat is more slowly digested and absorbed than all other foodstuffs. This is an important point for those wishing to reduce. The stomach feels full and contented for a longer period of time.

Liquid vegetable fats or oils should be used *instead of hard fats*. They should always be purchased at the health food store to assure freshness and should always be kept refrigerated after opening. Not less than one tablespoon a day should be taken, even when reducing. Take vitamin E when using the golden oils.

Powdered Milk, Also a Wonder Food

Powdered skim milk is free from animal fat and has many properties that classify it as another wonder food. It supplies you with a high biologic quality of protein, it is rich in calcium and riboflavin (vitamin B-2), and its vital nutritive factors are easily digested. Being a dry powder, it can be kept on hand at all times. It should be stored in a tightly sealed container in the dark to prevent it from becoming lumpy and also to keep it from losing its riboflavin content.

You can mix powdered milk for drinking, use it to fortify regular milk, or add it to your baking for calcium benefits to the whole family, as recommended by Dr. Hauser.

When recommending milk, remember that the refrigerated milk you buy from the store can be mucous forming. As with most of our foods, milk has been so changed from its natural state by additives and homogenizing that many doctors advise their patients not to use it.

Mrs. J. told me that she had a colonic and the doctor was very upset when he found her so full of mucus. He told her, "No more milk products!" She changed to raw vegetable and fruit juices and says she feels like a new person.

My husband could not drink even half a glass of milk without getting a terrible sinus headache. I found some raw, untreated milk in a health food store and had him drink a glass. He never had one bad reaction from the raw milk. We cannot improve on nature.

THE WONDER FOOD CALLED LECITHIN

We could not exist without lecithin (linoleic acid). This nutrient combines with proteins and cholesterol to form structures so basic that there is no life without them. One structure forms the membranes that enclose every living cell. If such a membrane is absent, weak, or faulty in structure, the contents of the cells leak out and the cells die. If the cells die, then the body dies.

Lecithin also forms myelin, a fatty protein substance that sheathes the major nerves of the body, including the spinal cord. If there is damage to this sheath, it can impair the mentality and be a cause of neurological symptoms, even the dread multiple sclerosis. It may be possible that atherosclerosis is also caused by a deficiency of lecithin.

Lecithin is said to regulate the coagulation of the blood so that it is neither too fast nor too slow. It guards against coronary thrombosis and strokes by preventing clotting, and it is also effective against ulcers, asthma and other allergic conditions, dental cavities, and acne and other skin disorders. (Lecithin is one of the building blocks of the teeth.)

Danger of Lecithin

Dr. Tappel tells us that lecithin can also be dangerous if taken without the antitoxin, vitamin E. It seems that this very necessary vitamin can become rancid within our bodies. Dr. Tappel states that rancid lecithin can cause damage to the "structural and functional components of the cell," so it is absolutely essential to take vitamin E, and bioflavonoid (found in garlic) as well, when you ingest lecithin. This proves that we do need balanced vitamins and minerals.

We are told of tests that were made on people of different ages who were suffering from loss of memory. When they were given thirty grams of lecithin, their memory improved, some as much as 25 percent. I knew that this is true—I tried it on myself and it did give me more mind power. Calcium (bone meal) should also be taken to balance any excess phosphorus from the lecithin.

THE IMPORTANCE OF VITAMIN A

Vitamin A is one of the easiest vitamins to obtain in the diet. It is not lost in cooking or storing and is generally present in the average American diet. Yet, nutritionists find that most people seem to be on the borderline of deficiency.

There are many symptoms of vitamin A deficiency, including night blindness and certain skin diseases.

All symptoms of vitamin A deficiency are quickly relieved by a sufficient amount being added to the diet, but several conditions keep the body from absorbing this vitamin, in which case you will need to ingest more of it. One way to make sure that you get enough vitamin A and vitamin D in your diet is to take cod liver oil daily. Even better, halibut liver oil is said to contain about a hundred times as much vitamin A as does cod liver oil.

I gave my children one teaspoon of cod liver oil the first thing in the morning every day from the time they were very young until they left home. I did not know it at that time, but I was doing the right thing by giving it to them on an empty stomach.

Vitamin A and Dry Skin

Dale Alexander, author of *Arthritis and Common Sense* tells us that dry skin is a warning sign that something is wrong within the body and it is crying for help. He tells us, "Your skin is the barometer of your health. It mirrors the condition of your whole body."

If you have dry skin, then you have much more than dry skin. You have dryness throughout your body. It is not merely a skin problem; it means that all parts of your body need lubrication. When you have a health problem, the first place it shows is in your skin.

This is why so many people who use reflex massage claim that all symptoms of dry skin disappear after massaging and pressing the buttons to all tender reflexes. They are using the method of reflexology to stimulate the organs and glands within the body that have been sending signals for help by causing dry skin. It means that your whole system is drying out. It means that you are beginning to age before your time. I will tell you more about dry skin and its importance to your health in Chapter 34, on beauty and your skin.

For now, remember the importance of cod liver oil, which lubricates the whole inner body. Mr. Alexander tells us the best way to take it is in a small amount of milk or orange juice one hour before you eat any food or four hours or more after you have eaten. Cod liver oil also gives you vitamin D.

To take cod liver oil, place one teaspoon of the oil in a small bottle, add about two ounces of milk, shake until foamy, and drink (on an empty stomach). Wait one hour before eating. This gives the intestines time to absorb and utilize the cod liver oil before the liver can grab it. If you can't take milk, orange juice may be used instead, but milk is really the best according to Mr. Alexander.

Although cod liver oil has a bad taste, my children never minded it, probably because they had taken it all of their lives. Now you can buy it in several flavors, which make it much easier to take. Be sure that it is fresh when you buy it and keep it in the refrigerator after you have opened it.

Insurance Refused Because of Good Health

After my son was married he decided to take out life insurance. After filling out the necessary papers and having an examination, he waited for the final policy but never received it. He discovered that the salesman was questioning a lot of his friends about him and his health. He asked the salesman why he was investigating his private life. The salesman replied: "I thought that you were trying to cover up some kind of an illness because in all my years of selling insurance I have never known anyone who was as healthy as you claim to be. You have never had any ailments besides the normal children's illnesses, and you've never been to a doctor in your life! It just didn't ring true. I couldn't believe it, so I had to try to prove what you told me." I believe now that the cod liver oil, along with a good natural diet, is the reason my family enjoys perfect health. Of course, since the discovery of reflexology, we all keep healthy and free from illnesses with the added conscientious use of reflex massage.

VITAMIN C, THE MIRACLE VITAMIN

Vitamin C is one of the miracle vitamins in use today. It is inexpensive and available in health food stores, drugstores, and even in grocery stores. Vitamin C is lauded for its wonderful healing power for nearly every illness, including heart disease, strokes, and arthritis.

When vitamin C was first brought to my attention, it was described as preventing and curing colds. I immediately started to use it to stop colds before they actually got started.

Vitamin C Cures Chronic Bronchitis

One day Mrs. G., a friend I was visiting, told me of her family's cold problems. Every winter they spent several weeks in the hospital with flu and congested lungs. Gene, about nine years old, had suffered with bronchitis all his life. I told her about vitamin C and its healing properties, especially for colds. She said she would try it. A few months later, I again went to visit Mrs. G. and she told me what happened with the vitamin C that she had bought. She said that she placed the bottle on the table, but no one took any of the tablets.

One day, Mrs. G. noticed that the vitamin bottle on the table was empty, so she asked Gene about this. He said that since she had told him, "They are good for you and will make you well," he figured he would take them all and get well all at once—and he did get well all at once!

The following winter was one of the worst for colds and flu. Mrs. G. told me that they had all spent weeks in the hospital with colds and

bronchial infections—but not Gene. He never had a cold or even a snif-
fle all winter long.

The next time I saw Gene he was in his twenties, and was a big,
healthy, strong man who had never had a recurrence of bronchitis since
the time he took the whole bottle of vitamin C.

I would not advise anyone to take an overdose of any vitamin, but in
clinical studies they are proving that megadoses of vitamins are the answer
to many puzzling health problems that modern medication will not cure.

Vitamins A and C reduce the damage smoking causes the body.
If you can't quit smoking, take more vitamins A and C.

The late Paavo Airola, a noted nutritionist, said that vitamin C is
involved in virtually all the functions of your body. It helps your body
to protect itself against every stress and every condition threatening
your health.

Dr. M. Higuchi, a Japanese researcher, tells us that his studies
show a definite relationship between vitamin C levels in the diet and
hormone production of the sex glands. He says that older people, particularly, need larger amounts of vitamin C to assure adequate sex hormone production.

When taking any vitamin or mineral tablets, I powder the tablets
for better assimilation. To do this, lay the tablet between two sheets
of waxed paper and crush with a hammer until it is powdered.
Sprinkle on food or put into a milk or a drink. I suggest that you
experiment on your own to find out how you like to take it best. Some
vitamins are available in powdered and liquid form, others are made
with natural flavors and are chewable.

GARLIC, A MIRACLE FOOD

I must not leave out the importance of garlic. It is known as a miracle vegetable. It has been used for thousands of years by various races
and civilizations. Early Egyptians and Hebrews considered garlic a
food endowed with divine properties—and it really is. Garlic is rich in
several food chemicals as well as vitamins A, B, C, and D. (Vitamin D
is the sunshine vitamin so necessary for existence.) It is also rich in sulfur and iodine. All these help to stimulate the liver and kidneys, eliminate worms from children and pets, and relieve rheumatic and arthritic conditions and many other ailments.

Garlic also contains bioflavonoid, which is needed when you are taking the wonder food lecithin. (Combined garlic and lecithin capsules are now available.)

I have proved the marvelous healing properties of garlic in my personal life. As a child, I was always ill. When we moved to California, I played with some children who were eating bread and butter and garlic. I had never heard of garlic before. When they gave me a bit of their garlic bread, I loved it! I couldn't get enough of it! I ate it constantly, my family putting up with my bad odor. I don't know how long I was on a garlic binge, but I never had a sick spell again. I had a cast-iron stomach and still do.

My mother had high blood pressure until a doctor told her to eat lots of garlic, which she did. She took the little bulbs like pills quite often for a few years. She never suffered with high blood pressure again, and she lived into her nineties.

When I went to Alaska, I went to a wonderful doctor for a physical examination. When I went back for the results of the tests she had taken, she took my blood pressure and was surprised to see that it was a little high. She said that she didn't believe it was anything to be concerned about. I told her that, usually, when I thought I had high blood pressure, I ate garlic. She whirled around on her stool and looked at me a moment. I thought, "Boy, I sure said the wrong thing this time." But the doctor pointed her finger at me and said, "You just keep taking that garlic." She knew the value of natural remedies and wasn't afraid to say so. I could write an entire book on the value of garlic to your health.

Garlic is also excellent for pets.

Along with garlic, onions are also an excellent blood purifier and are helpful to your health in other ways. Include plenty of garlic and onions in your diet every day, preferably raw.

THE VALUE OF HERBS

I am not going to discuss herbs in this book. There are many fine books already on the market by noted herbalists. I do believe that you should understand a little about their importance to your health and well-being, however. "For every illness there is an herb." I know that this is true. I have used herbs for years. Herbs cured my late husband of his heart trouble. They were introduced to us by Dewy Conway, an Indian herb doctor in Chico, California.

When you make herb tea, *do not boil it*. Honey and lemon may be added if desired. My favorite herb tea is sage and rosemary. This is good to strengthen many parts of the body. It has a cool fresh taste and leaves the stomach feeling clean and refreshed. A little peppermint may be added if desired. This herb tea is very relaxing, so it is a good drink to take before going to bed. Ask the salesperson at your health food store about herbs and their uses.

DANGERS OF TOO MUCH PROTEIN

Eating lots of protein used to be recommended. But I have always contended that we eat too much protein.

Consider the health and longevity of the Hunzas. A group of people living in the Himalayas in a valley at the base of Mt. Everest. In the last few years, several of our leading biologically and nutritionally oriented doctors have traveled to the valley of the Hunzas and studied the people and their diets. Their diet consists mostly of vegetables and fruit, with very low protein consumption, and they enjoy health and vitality past their one-hundredth birthdays. We stand in envy and awe and wonder what happened to *us*.

The Max Planck Institute in Germany and the Russian Institute for Nutritional Research tell us that too much protein in the diet is extremely dangerous and can cause health disturbances and serious diseases.

We hear about women dying from going on a high-protein weight-reducing diet. I can tell you of a personal experience with a liquid high-protein diet. You should know that I will not recommend anything that I do not try myself first. This powdered protein sounded good—it was made up of all natural grains, nuts, and so on, but before I would recommend it, I had to try it myself. I did—and it nearly killed me! In three days, I started to feel bad; then, I developed terrible pains in my back muscles; before I realized what was happening, the tightness in my back muscles continued on around my body to my lungs, so I could hardly breathe. The pain was continuous, but I was able to control it, somewhat, with the reflex clamps and the reflex comb, massaging the endocrine glands reflexes. If I had not gone to an excellent chiropractor, who is also a naturopathic doctor, I am sure I would have died. I can certainly understand why so many people die who go on these high-protein diets and then, in desperation, turn to their medical doctors who may not understand nutrition and are helpless, not knowing what to do. I was put on a lemon juice diet.

The common belief that only animal proteins are complete and that all vegetable proteins are incomplete is false. Too much protein can cause a severe deficiency of magnesium and vitamins B-6 and B-3; also, too much animal protein may be the cause of such diseases as arthritis, osteoporosis, and heart disease. It can also cause mental disorders, particularly schizophrenia. Too much animal protein leads to premature aging caused by a chemical imbalance, overacidity in tissues, intestinal putrefaction, constipation, and degeneration of vital organs.

Dr. Nathan Pritikin tells us why a high-protein diet is harmful. When your protein intake exceeds approximately 16 percent of your caloric intake of about 3,200 calories daily, you go into a negative mineral balance. He tells us that almost everyone on the average American diet is in a negative mineral balance. This means that your body is actually losing its precious stores of important minerals such as calcium, iron, zinc, phosphorus, and magnesium. Even though some people take mineral supplements, it does not always remedy this loss of life-sustaining minerals.

Too much protein along with sugar and honey can raise insulin levels dangerously, and it can raise uric acid levels, creating a risk of gout.

When tested on animals, it was learned that when the protein was reduced the animals developed a greater resistance to certain blood and breast cancers. When protein in rodent feed was cut from 26 percent to 4 percent, both rats and mice lived longer and healthier lives.

ELECTRICAL VIBRATIONS FROM LIVE FOOD AFFECT YOUR HEALTH

Any cooked food is dead food. How can you have healthy live cells if you feed them dead foods? The sure and proven way to keep healthy and stay young longer is to eat mostly live foods—raw or lightly steamed vegetables, fresh fruits, seeds, nuts, grains, and especially sprouted seeds like alfalfa or bean sprouts.

Live food has a vibratory rate that generates life! Take, for instance, calcium found in chalk—it has little life vibration that we can use. Then, take the calcium found in cabbage or turnip greens. This calcium has a vibrant life, biochemical activity. This calcium is life giving. This holds true in all the live foods that grow. When they are overcooked or sit on the shelves of the market, they lose some of the electrical vibratory life energy.

This electrical vibratory life is created through the activity of sun, air, and water. It takes a living thing to keep another living thing alive.

I recommend reading the national health magazine *Health Freedom News*, The National Health Federation, P.O. Box 688, Monrovia, California 91016. This is a very informative magazine that dares tell the truth about health.

CHAPTER 12

Why Drinking Water and Deep Breathing Are Critical to Reflexology

We all know that we need oxygen and water to live. We cannot live more than a few days without water, and no more than a few minutes without air. Our body's living cells need both water and oxygen to function.

THE WONDERS OF PURE WATER

Our body is 70 percent water. It is the most abundant substance of our being. Every part of the body needs and depends on water. Our entire system requires water to function properly, to lubricate our joints, to regulate body temperature and to aid digestion. Water is needed by the kidneys to flush wastes, and by the blood to help carry nutrients and oxygen to body cells so that we will be able to maintain beautiful hair and soft moist skin. Muscles must have fluids or they will become weak and shrivel away. And we cannot forget how imperative water is to washing out excess fats.

Why You Need to Drink Water When Using Reflexology

When your body has a shortage of water, the blood draws it from the tissues and cells, and a state of dehydration takes place. When this happens, the body's performance suffers. It is better to drink too much water rather than not enough. Your kidneys will readily release any excess water. Reflexology aids nature in cleaning the body of toxins and impurities through the elimination of liquid wastes, as it balances and revitalizes the whole system.

When you have a cold, you know the importance of drinking more liquids to flush the germs from your system. The body must have enough water for both structural existence and to function properly every day. Absence of water in the body's cells may hinder the response of stimulation through reflexology. So you will want to drink plenty of pure water.

Reflexologist Explains "WATER IS THE CONDUCTOR"

At a gathering in Kansas, I had the opportunity to meet with a fellow reflexologist, Zackery Brinkerhoff, who has a sixty-year history of reflexology success in his family. He told us about one of his clients, who at first did not respond to reflexology, or any other natural therapy. He felt totally helpless and mystified until one day he attended a seminar at the University of Colorado, and there he learned how important water consumption is to the body's healing process. He told us "water is the conductor of the electrical stimulus that is created through reflexology, absence of liquid in the cells of the nerve structures hinders the movement of the nerve signal. Hence . . . no response."

Brinkerhoff later contacted his client to tell her the good news and she confirmed that a medical report revealed that she was *severely dehydrated*. He then told us "As she began to drink more water, her body returned to a normal state of hydration and responded to reflexology in a measurable and observable way and she improved accordingly.

HOW TO PURIFY YOUR WATER
FOR SAFE DRINKING

You must be sure that the water you drink is safe. If you are uncertain about the water where you are, disinfect the water and kill any infectious bacteria by bringing the water to a full boil for five minutes; after it cools, put the water into a container and shake it vigorously. This will improve the flat taste and oxygenate it.

To add energy to your drinking water, take the container and swirl it in a spiral motion, so that the water moves in a circular action.

This will regenerate the water with natural electricity. As we drink pure clean water, our bodies will develop new strength and energy, because water supports all living things.

DEEP BREATHING AND REFLEXOLOGY GO HAND-IN-HAND

Reflexology and deep breathing will do wonders for your health. Using this combination you will improve your immune power and balance your blood pressure. Your entire cardiovascular and respiratory systems need oxygen. Have you ever tried to burn a fire without air? It will not happen. And it is the same with your body; it must have oxygen from the air you breathe to maintain vibrant health and energy. You will discover that with the use of reflexology and deep breathing, your circulation and mental abilities will improve.

This combination also will help you to develop body awareness. As you learn more about reflexology and proper breathing, you will focus on various parts of the body and learn more about yourself.

Breathe Your Way to Good Health

Every part of our body is composed of many trillions of tiny cells. It is through breathing that oxygen is carried to these cells by the bloodstream. No red blood cells can be built without oxygen.

A single cell could be compared to a toy balloon. Inflate it with air and it is firm, young, ready to lift into the skies. But let the balloon develop a leak, and it soon loses its tone, begins to shrivel, finally sinking wearily to the ground.

It is the same way with an individual, minute body cell. Unless provided with sufficient oxygen, it becomes depleted, tired, and lifeless. As a result, the whole body begins to lose its youthfulness and vitality.

Oxygen More Important than Food

Actually oxygen is more important than food; without enough oxygen, food cannot be changed into nourishment the body demands. One can exist without food for a considerable time. But without air, life ceases in minutes.

Blood feeds cells, organs, glands, nerves, tissues, hair, teeth, bones, skin, and nails. If we have healthy oxygenated blood, we can count on a body resistant to infection and illness. The need for proper breathing has its bearing on all the activities of the body. Deep breathing can be compared to a thorough spring housecleaning. A poorly ventilated room feels stuffy and has an unpleasant odor. The same is true of a body in need of oxygen.

DEEP BREATHING EXERCISES

Knowing the correct way to do deep breathing exercises is critical to good health. Eventually, with practice, it will come naturally and almost unconsciously. To most people it will be a new and novel experience, sending fresh oxygen to every part of the body.

Correct posture is important when doing deep breathing exercises. If you sit on the floor, do so in a cross-legged position so the spine is very straight. You may use a straight-backed chair instead, or if one has to remain in bed, try to have the back as straight as possible. This is most important.

With back straight and mouth closed, slowly start drawing in a breath, feeling it along your throat. Forget that you have nostrils. The breath must come into the throat. You will feel it on the top portion of the upper throat. It will make a slight hissing sound.

Instead of this air going into the top of the lungs as in normal breathing, it is being sucked down to the very bottom. You will feel the rib cage expand from the bottom. When you believe you have filled your lungs, let the air out slowly, mouth closed, air pressed against the top of the upper throat. This slight hissing sound will be heard again, probably only by you.

Stay relaxed. Breathe very slowly, letting out air from the upper part of the chest first, and going downward until lungs are empty. It will seem awkward at first, and possibly difficult, but gradually it will become second nature.

Now try it again, putting your hands on each side of the ribs, feeling them expand as you breathe deep down from bottom up. As the air is slowly expelled, feel the ribs go down from the upper part, pulling in the stomach slightly. In ordinary breathing, the chest does not rise.

This deep breathing should not be done more than two breaths at a time the first day. You might like to do it in the morning, in the afternoon and in the evening. It can be gradually increased, doing three at a time the second day.

This will take practice and time, but it's well worth the effort if you truly want to be young and healthy for the rest of your life.

CHAPTER 13

How Reflexology Helps the Colon

I am wondering how many of you realize how important the colon (large intestine) is to your general well-being and health. While I visited the office of a naturopathic doctor recently, I saw some pictures of diseases and abnormalities of the colon. They were horrifying. Even I did not realize how completely the colon can become diseased, even while the body keeps on functioning. (Not comfortably, though, for sure.)

FATAL ILLNESS CAN BEGIN IN THE COLON

The colon is a good sewage system, but by neglect and abuse it becomes a cesspool. It can be the cause of more physical human misery and suffering, mental and moral, than any other known source.

The colon takes up a large space in your body. It carries off all the waste matter that is left from the food and drink that you send into your stomach by way of the mouth.

What happens when you don't empty your garbage can for a few days? What if you emptied just part of the garbage? What would happen to the garbage that didn't get emptied for months, yes, even years, as you kept adding to the waste? You can buy a new garbage can every so often, but do you want to have to buy a new colon? Some people have to, you know! If you could have seen the pictures of the insides of some diseased colons, as I did, you wouldn't let one day go

132

by before you started to do something about helping your colon to maintain or regain its normal health.

TROUBLES OF THE COLON

Notice the colon in Diagram 10. See how large it is and how much of the body it occupies. Can you picture the whole inside of this organ literally covered with sores, all inflamed and abscessed and unable to carry off the waste material that you are still forcing into it? No wonder there is such a high rate of colon cancer today.

While your colon is filled with pollution, your bloodstream is drawing some of this poison and feeding it back into the body.

Remember that *every cell of the body is served by the blood*. It nourishes the cells, replaces "worn-out" parts, and carries away waste products. If you have an infection in the body, such as infected teeth, the doctors fear it will poison the rest of your body, in some way causing arthritis or other related diseases. How many of you are letting your blood feed your body on decayed sewage from your colon? Do not wait until it is too late! Start to repair it now with reflex massage. I will also tell you of other remedies to heal a sick colon if it is not completely beyond repair.

After studying pictures of diseased colons, I asked a doctor, "How can people live with such terrible colons?" He said, "The body is a wonderful system beyond our understanding and is able to do marvelous jobs repairing itself."

USING REFLEXOLOGY FOR THE COLON

First let us try a little test to see if the colon reflexes are tender or sore. Since we are just testing, let us try the colon reflexes on the hand. The colon reflex is almost straight across the middle of the hand. See Diagram 3.

Take the thumb of the right hand or a massaging device and start pressing it into the pad in the middle of the left hand. See Photos 31 and 34. Starting below the pad under the little finger, search for tender spots as you work the thumb or a massaging device across the center of the palm until you come to the area between the thumb and the forefinger. If you find a tender reflex on your way across the palm, massage it for a moment or hold pressure on it to the count of seven.

Change hands, and with the thumb of the left hand, press and massage across the center of the palm of the right hand as you search out tender spots that indicate malfunction elsewhere in the body. This does not necessarily mean that it is only the colon reflexes that are giving you the warning signal, for there are several reflexes crowded into the palms of the hands. See Photo "D."

Go on to the reflexes in the pad below the thumb. This area also has reflexes to several other parts of the body, so if it has any tender spots in it, be sure to massage them out. In many cases, a reflex device will probably be helpful here, especially the magic reflex massager or the reflex hand probe.

Go to the web between the thumb and forefinger. Using the thumb and forefinger of the right hand or a reflex device, pinch and massage this web on the left hand. See Photos 35 and 37 and Photo "C." This is another area that holds reflexes to several parts of the body, so if there are any tender spots, be sure to massage every one of them out. Remember that we must have the whole body in harmony to bring it into perfect balance and health.

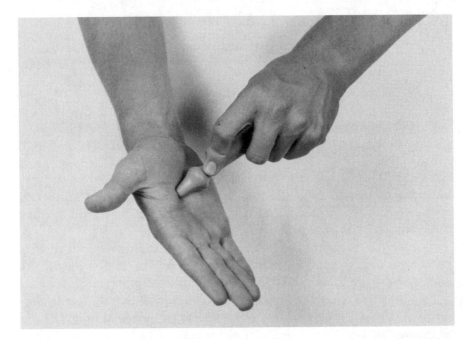

Photo "D": Using hand probe to work the reflexes to several parts of the body, including the colon and intestines.

Change hands and massage the web of the right hand. Never do one side of the body without doing the other. This would cause an unbalanced condition of the whole electrical nervous system.

We are going to massage another area where the reflexes also go to many parts of the body. From the web that you have just been massaging, press the thumb on up into the fleshy part of the hand between the bones of the thumb and the forefinger. See Diagrams 6A and 6D. In this area, search for tender reflexes in the center and also along the bones of the thumb and the forefinger. In other chapters, you will be referred to this same reflex area for various ailments.

Other Colon Reflexes

Now, we will go to the forefinger for another reflex to the colon. Press the finger starting at the nail, searching for a tender reflex. Work all the way up the arm as in Photo 41. There is also a reflex to the colon just under the lower lip.

I do not want to give you too many reflex points to work on as it gets confusing when there are too many to remember. Since the function of this organ is so important to the well-being of the whole body, I want you to do everything that you can to get it into as perfect condition as possible and then keep it that way.

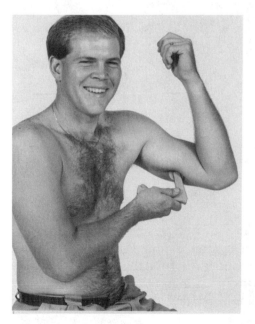

Photo 41: Position for massaging the many reflexes in the arm with the reflex roller massager. Laughter will stimulate the body's circulation and release tensions.

Massaging the Feet

Now, we will go to the colon reflexes in the feet. If it is difficult to lift your foot high enough to work on it, I suggest the reflex foot massager. See Photos 42 and 43. It is perfect for massaging all the reflexes on the bottom of the feet, especially the reflex to the colon. I use this reflex massager quite often while watching television in the evening. It keeps my body in perfect order while it relaxes the nervous system. Don't use it for too long at a time at first.

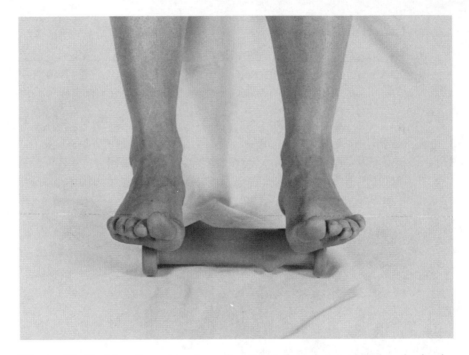

Photo 42: Position for using the reflex foot massager to energize the healing life force into most parts of the body.

For those of you who have your feet up where you can work on them, take your thumb or a reflex device, and start at the center or waistline of the foot. See Diagram 5 and Photos 44 and 45. Using a pressing, rolling motion, go across the foot toward the reflexes to the spine, then continue to massage on down the inside of the spine reflexes, all the time searching for tender reflexes.

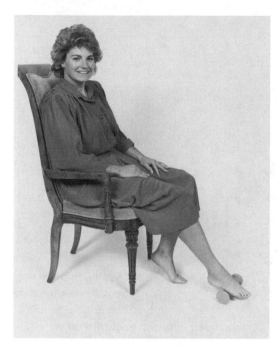

Photo 43: Shows comfortable position while using the reflex foot massager to help nature rejuvenate the body naturally.

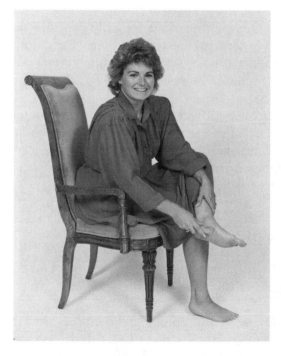

Photo 44: Shows how to use the reflex roller massager on the feet to help the back and the uterus.

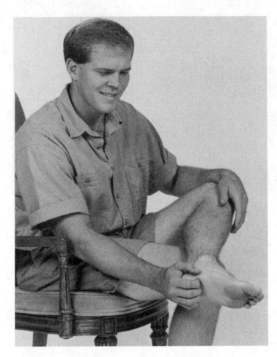

Photo 45: Position for massaging the reflexes under the heel pad to relieve painful problems in the lower half of the body.

When you find tender areas, either hold a steady pressure on them or massage them. If you are having trouble with the colon, you will find some of these spots almost too sore to touch. Start out gently at first, and as the soreness becomes less, you can increase the pressure.

Massage in this manner on both feet. Massage down the outer side of the foot toward the heel. You cannot be sure if it is the colon or other organs sending out the pain signal as you massage over certain areas. Don't let this concern you. Just keep in mind that where congestion exists, disease will result, so massage it out.

OTHER REMEDIES FOR THE COLON

Since the colon is one of the most important organs in your body, I will tell you a few more things to do along with the reflexology treatments to keep it healthy.

The most common disease of the colon, diverticulosis, strikes one of every three people over age sixty. Before 1900, this disease was almost unknown. Then diets were rich in whole grains, fruits, and vegetables, all good sources of fiber. Fiber, the indigestible portion of food, passes unaltered into the lower bowel, adding bulk to the stool and helping keep the bowels in good working order. We hear much today about bran, for instance. One of the best sources of bran fiber is the husk of wheat and other grains. White flour, meat, dairy products, and sugar are low in fiber. Low-fiber diets create small, hard stools. When these reach the colon, that organ has to clamp down and squeeze unnaturally hard to force them through. A lifetime of this kind of overwork weakens the muscles of the colon, causing small pouches to protrude out the lining wall of the colon. These pouches are called diverticula; if they are present, you have diverticulosis. When bran fiber was added to the diet of those suffering from this malfunction of the colon, 90 percent of the patients were relieved of the disease. Also relieved were such symptoms as bloody stools, constipation, and nausea.

Do you understand why I give you this advice along with the reflexology massage? Things of nature work together to create a perfect balance, and fiber is one of nature's healing foods. We might refer to it as a scrub brush as it passes through the alimentary canal. See Diagram 9.

SAUERKRAUT, A HEALING AGENT

Sauerkraut is a health-giving, vitamin-producing food that has been a boon to man for centuries. Sauerkraut regulates the digestive processes, overcomes vitamin and mineral deficiencies, and stimulates the body to longer life. It provides the body with all the benefits of green and leafy vegetables at all times of the year besides adding other qualities that other vegetables do not have.

Sauerkraut supplies lime, iron, bone and blood builders, and other vital vitamins and minerals. It is a fermented product made from cabbage. To certain peoples of the world, sauerkraut means health and an extraordinary sense of well-being; it is an economical and satisfying food. It is an easily digestible vegetable that combines, in a most savory manner, with other foods and—by the experience of many centuries—also is a food that seems to prolong life.

You may wonder why I am writing so much about sauerkraut in this chapter on the colon. It is a perfect food to help heal problems in the colon. I know of no other natural food that can take its place.

It is a proven fact that some ailments are caused by the large amounts of harmful bacteria that reside in the large intestine. These intestinal microbes manufacture poisons that spread throughout the body. These microbes are produced by the waste products of the food we eat.

According to Elie Metchnikoff of the Pasteur Institute, "In arteriosclerosis in the cases of patients who do not suffer from special diagnosed causes, the blame must fall on the innumerable microbes that swarm in our intestines and poison us."

Metchnikoff claimed that, "The presence of large numbers of lactic acid bacilli will interfere with the development of the putrefactive bacteria."

How Sauerkraut Helps

This is the role that sauerkraut plays in helping your colon heal itself: it is a natural lactic acid food that overcomes harmful germs in the large intestines (used in place of dangerous drugs) and it helps relieve constipation, which is largely the cause of colon problems. Sauerkraut is an excellent regulator and a natural laxative.

A Friend Is Helped

A friend of mine said that she had to give up square dancing because of colon problems. I said, "Why don't you eat sauerkraut?" She was surprised at my suggestion, but she did say she would try it. (She wouldn't try reflexology as she couldn't understand how it works.) I didn't see her for several months after that. I went back to the dance one night and she came up to me and thanked me for making her well. I had forgotten the earlier incident, so I didn't know what she was talking about. I thought she was talking about reflexology, but then she began to explain to me about taking the sauerkraut. She had eaten sauerkraut every day; her colon had gotten well, and she had been dancing every night since.

Sauerkraut Helps Many Organs

It is not only because of its varied vitamin content that I recommend sauerkraut in the diet, but also because it is rich in mineral substances.

It contains large quantities of calcium, sulfur, chlorine, and iodine in a natural form.

Because of its minerals, sauerkraut is a valuable aid in the preservation of teeth, gums, hair, and bones. We know that sauerkraut acts as a blood cleanser and relieves constipation. It also aids in the function of the kidneys and the bladder and is a helpful agent in cases of functional heart trouble.

Try to include sauerkraut in your menu every day. It is good cooked with pork and garlic. It makes a delicious dressing combined with apples and onions and stuffed in a duck or a chicken. It is good to use in salads, cold or heated, with oil and garlic powder added. If it is too sour for you, add honey to taste. Eat applesauce with sauerkraut; it is delicious. Drink sauerkraut juice to help in a reducing diet. I would suggest a daily intake of sauerkraut or juice as a preventive measure against general ill health.

ENEMAS FOR PROBLEMS IN THE COLON

Some doctors advise us to take enemas; others advise us not to take enemas. Here we are going to tell you how to take enemas to help a sick colon, and we are going to use one of our wonder foods, *blackstrap molasses*. Yes! An enema taken with this black magic has cured abscesses in the colon. I know this is true because it was my colon that was healed. This was in the days before I knew very much about natural healing. I knew for a long time that I had an abscess in my colon. It would become very painful at times, and sometimes it would break and drain. I never went to doctors unless I was having a baby. They always wanted to operate on me for something when I did go, so I quit going. I continually studied natural healing methods and got a small book about blackstrap molasses. It said to use two tablespoons of the molasses to a quart of water for an enema, so I started to take the enemas and felt better almost immediately. Soon the abscess started to drain; it looked like a boil draining with pus and blood. I kept taking the molasses enemas for a few more days, and I never had any trouble with the colon again.

The Key to Locked Bowels

Mrs. A. tells of a day a few years back when she became very constipated. A doctor told her that she had "locked bowels" and that they would have to operate. She called her sister, who was a nurse, and told her what the doctor had said. "Don't you do anything until I get there," the sister told her. When her sister arrived the next day, she asked for some blackstrap molasses. (This should be from a health food store only.) She prepared an enema with it, making it quite strong. She gave her sister the enemas, one after another, until she finally got the bowel to release the blockage, and her sister was saved from a dangerous operation. Mrs. A. claims that blackstrap molasses and her sister saved her life.

One day, I was visiting a chiropractor who was always interested in talking about health. We would go into his office and talk for hours. I have learned many things from this wonderful man who was interested in all types of natural healing. He told me of the time that he worked in a clinic that specialized in colon diseases. They had a special formula that they used on all colon patients to cure problems of the colon without operations. I am giving this formula to you as I have given it to others who have had success with it. Keep in mind that if you do not get results in a few days from any of the methods that I have given you, see a doctor—a good naturopath, if possible.

Formula for a Sick Colon

2 oz. chlorophyll, liquid or powder
1 tablespoon glycerine
1 teaspoon Gold Seal (liquid tincture, if available)
4 oz. witch hazel
8 oz. stale beer (12 hours old)

Mix all ingredients and use as an enema. Retain or hold this enema one half-hour. Do this at least once a day or more often for two days. If your problem is severe, extend the treatment to five or six days. Then take the enemas every other day. Take daily: acidophilus, yogurt, and sauerkraut every day.

What to Eat to Keep Your Colon Healthy

It has been proven in clinical tests that people who eat a lot of foods from the cabbage family have much more freedom from all diseases of the colon than do those who eat none or very little of the cabbage plants. In addition to sauerkraut, these include broccoli, brussels sprouts, and cauliflower. If you are inclined to have colon problems, start including these good-for-you vegetables in your diet.

CHAPTER 14

How Reflexology Strengthens the Liver

The liver is the largest gland in the body. It weighs about three pounds in an adult and has, at all times, about one quarter of all the blood in the body circulating through it.

The liver performs many tasks: it is a great filter and it is a natural antiseptic and purgative device. It manufactures bile, which the intestines use to digest fats and prevent constipation. It helps to supply some of the substances for making blood and it also stores sugar.

HAND AND FOOT REFLEXES

Since the liver is such a large organ, you will massage a larger area than usual. The reflexes to the liver are on the right hand and the right foot. Place the thumb of the left hand on the pad of the right hand or foot, just below the little finger or little toe. See Diagrams 3 and 5. Press and roll this area searching for tender spots. When you find them, massage them for about ten counts. In many cases, you will probably need a reflex device like the magic massager or the hand massager. The liver is sometimes stubborn in its response to healing methods. Be persistent in your efforts to open up the channels to allow the electric life forces to surge in full power to the ailing liver.

HOW THE LIVER RESISTS

Though the liver sometimes seems to resist our efforts to help bring it back to its natural full capacity of work, it is one gland that can replace parts of itself. Remember its importance to your complete health, and massage all the reflexes to the liver.

If you have a very sluggish liver, start out with a light massage the first few times. You can expect different reactions from this treatment of the liver. If it is very sensitive and you do have a severe reaction, don't massage the liver reflexes for a few days. Give nature a chance to throw off excess poisons and adjust itself to the increased circulation that the electrical life force has put into motion.

There is also a very important liver reflex on the large pad of the right thumb, and one on the right big toe as well. This is the same area that you worked when you worked on the reflex to the heart on the left hand and foot. Massage this pad very thoroughly, and if you find tender reflexes here, remember our motto, "If it hurts, work it out."

Go to the web between the thumb and the forefinger. Pinch and squeeze the reflexes in this area. If you find any tender spots, massage them out. Remember that they also open up the electrical channels to other parts of the body. See Photos 35 and 36.

While you are on the web, with the thumb on top of the hand, work the thumb right up between the bones of the thumb and the forefinger. See Diagram 6D. Press and squeeze this whole area. If it is easier for you to use the forefinger on the top of the hand instead of the thumb, then do it that way. Massage along the bones on both sides as you search for tender spots.

LIVER REFLEXES ALSO HELP
THE GALLBLADDER

The gallbladder is lodged on the under surface of the right lobe of the liver. It is a pear-shaped vibromuscular receptacle for the bile. This is also the receptable where the very painful hardened masses called gallstones are found. I have received letters from many people telling me of how reflex massage on the hands and feet has dissipated gallstones after a few treatments. It is not known whether the treatments so relaxed the gall duct that they passed off or whether the stones dissolved. If you find any of these reflex buttons to be tender, massage them until all soreness is gone. Do not try to rub out all the tenderness at one time. Give nature time to relieve this congestion. Remember, it took a long time for the body to get into this condition, so give it time to perform its own miracle of healing. The channels of the electrical life forces are opened when you press and massage these special reflex buttons to the liver and gallbladder.

Location of the Gallbladder Reflexes

Notice on Diagrams 7 and 8 that the reflex buttons to the liver are just below the ribs on the right side, and the gallbladder reflexes are located just below these buttons. With your middle finger, gently press in this area. Both fingers may be used simultaneously once you have located the reflex buttons. Remember that the liver covers a large area and you may find more than one "ouch" button. Hold a steady pressure on any tender reflex button that you find. Start just at the right of the navel and gently press, working over to your right side. Hold each tender reflex gently to the count of seven.

Now use the method described earlier in this book. Lay your hand flat on this whole area and in a clockwise motion roll the hand about three times over the whole right side. With all five fingers pressed together, place one or both hands just under the rib cage and vibrate or jiggle them. Continue this vibration until you have covered the whole liver area. With the flat of the right hand or both hands, lightly tap the whole liver area. Tapping with a wire brush here also will give you a feeling of renewed energy and health. The metal in the teeth of the brush adds to the power of the electrical energy.

HEAD REFLEXES TO THE LIVER

If you want to further stimulate the liver, look at Diagram 12 to see the reflexes to the internal organs which include the liver. They are located on the top of the head. Use pressure on each of these reflexes, holding to a slow count of about three. These will also be stimulated when you use the tapping method with the fingers or the wire brush as shown in Photos 10 and 11.

Now we turn to the reflexes in the ears. The ears contain reflexes to the whole body. Since it is difficult to pinpoint each reflex in such a small area, just massage the whole ear, searching for special "ouch" spots. Whatever this tender reflex is connected to, it is giving you a cry for help, so give it a few moments of massage by pinching and pulling on the whole ear. See Diagram 15 and Photos 18, 19, and 20.

CHAPTER 15

How Reflexology Helps the Pancreas and the Spleen

HELPING THE PANCREAS

The pancreas is one of the major balancing mechanisms of your metabolism. It is the maker of insulin, which lowers the sugar in the bloodstream (while adrenaline from your adrenal glands raises it).

I want to give you a warning. If you have diabetes, you could increase your body's natural supply of insulin when you massage the reflexes to the pancreas. Several times I have had people come to me after a treatment to ask if reflex massage could make a difference in the amount of insulin they need to take. One man said he had to cut his insulin by 50 percent after taking two treatments.

The pancreas lies just below the stomach. See Diagrams 7, 9, and 10. Study Diagram 7 to find a reflex button on the left side of the body. When you are massaging the reflexes to the pancreas, use the push-button method by pressing with the middle finger or all fingers. Starting on the left side below the ribs, press and hold for three seconds. Then, move an inch toward the center of the body and press again. Follow this procedure across the body to a little above the navel. If you find an "ouch" spot, press and hold it several times.

In Diagram 12, notice that there are reflex buttons near the outer edges on the top of the head. Press these areas to see if there is tenderness. You will probably stimulate these reflexes as you go over

147

the head with the fists and the wire brush as explained in the chapter on reflexes in the head, but test them out anyway.

A Facial Reflex

While you are looking at Diagram 12, notice the reflex button just above the lip. Test this for tenderness also. See Photo 46.

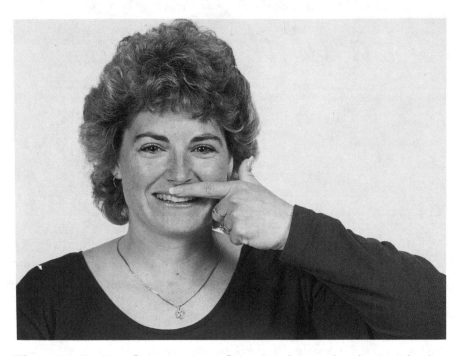

Photo 46: Position for massaging reflexes to spleen and endocrine glands to stimulate beauty and health. Also press and hold to stop a nosebleed and stifle a sneeze.

Reflexes in Hands and Feet

I cannot tell you often enough of the importance of the reflexes located in the hands and the feet. Many illnesses have been overcome by no other method than massaging the reflexes in the feet and the hands. Pain from most causes has been stopped within seconds by pressing certain reflex buttons located in these areas.

Look at Diagram 2 to see how the reflexes to the pancreas are located across the foot. Use the thumb, or the reflex roller if it is easier for you, to massage clear across the left foot and part way across the right foot. See Photos 42 and 43. As you work the pancreas reflexes, you will be covering the reflexes to several other glands as well. If you find this particular area of the pancreas especially tender, massage it out.

This technique also holds true for the reflexes in the hands. Use the same technique to work the reflexes to the pancreas by massaging across the left hand and also the right hand as you did on the feet. As you can see in Diagram 3, the reflexes in the hands are crowded one on top of the other. As you massage in this area, you are sending a charge of electrical healing force to many organs and glands in the body that are far removed from the area being massaged. This is why the magic massager gets such fantastic results when used conscientiously.

HELPING THE SPLEEN

Now let us look at the spleen. Notice in Diagram 10 that the spleen is located over part of the pancreas. The reflex to this little gland is just under or below the pad of the little toe near the heart reflex on the left foot and also on the left hand just below the pad of the little finger. See Diagrams 3 and 5.

Use the same technique to work this little reflex as you did for the pancreas. If you find an "ouch" spot in this reflex to the spleen, you might be anemic. This will give you a warning to have your blood checked. Anemia is caused by lack of iron in the blood and can cause serious trouble if neglected for a long period of time. You may also need folic acid. By massaging this reflex to the spleen, you will be opening up channels allowing the electric force to bring natural health into the spleen.

CHAPTER 16

Reflexology to Help Ailing Kidneys and Bladder

HELPING THE KIDNEYS

The kidney is another important organ of the body. When the kidneys fail to function, the body also stops functioning, so we can see that it is very important to keep the kidneys at top performance at all times. In this day of poisoned air, poisoned foods, and poisoned water, the kidneys have a very heavy work load trying to filter out all these toxins.

I have had friends die within a few days after being taken to the hospital for kidney problems. The doctors began to administer large doses of antibiotics and other drugs to fight off infections. The kidneys began to malfunction in the first place because they could not handle the impurities of the body; then, when they were flooded with massive doses of toxic poisons, they just collapsed.

Testing Kidney Reflexes

Notice in Diagram 5 that the kidney reflexes are located just a little above the center line, near the middle of the foot. Press on this reflex. If it is tender, you will know there is not enough circulation of the energy life force going to the kidneys. Massage this area a few times. It may be very tender. If you have thick soles or calluses on your feet, you may need a reflex device such as the little hand reflex massager.

The roller massager and also the foot massager work well here. See Photo 47. When massaging the reflexes to the kidneys, use caution and do not massage them very long at a time, not over thirty seconds at first. Remember, when you massage all the reflexes, you are releasing a lot of poison into the system and the kidneys have to work harder to get rid of it. So give them just a little help in the beginning.

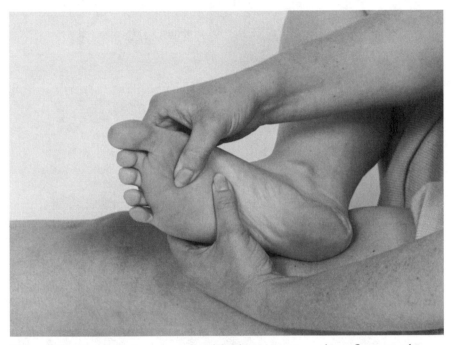

Photo 47: Shows how to use the thumbs to massage the reflexes to the kidney and thymus glands in the feet.

Now look to the hands. On Diagram 3 see where the reflexes are located in the center of the hands. Press and massage the kidney reflexes in the hands as you did on the feet. See Photos 31 and 34. When you use the magic reflex massager (Photo 48), you will naturally massage the kidney reflexes as you press the little fingers of the magic massager into all the reflexes in the hands. Placing clamps on the thumb and first two fingers will help kidneys and bladder. See Photo 49.

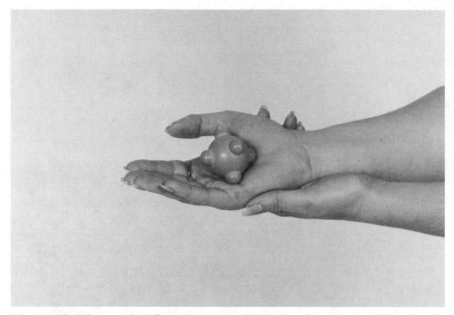

Photo 48: The magic reflex massager, which stimulates most of the glands and organs in the body.

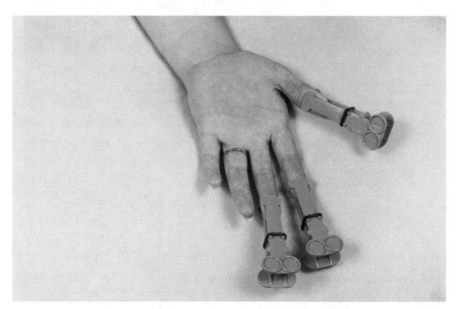

Photo 49: Shows reflex clamp on the first, second, and third fingers of the left hand to anesthetize zones 1, 2, and 3 of the body. See Diagram 16 on page 54.

Body Reflexes for the Kidneys

Remember, malfunction of the kidneys affects the bladder and sex glands, so when you massage the reflexes to the kidneys, you also activate the sex glands and bladder. See in Diagrams 7 and 8 that the kidney reflexes are near the sides of the body. With the fingers, press into this area, which is in the soft space between the rib cage and the hip bone. This position will place your thumbs on the soft area of the back. Now, slide the thumbs a little more toward the spine, feeling for tender spots. This is about where your kidneys are located. Press and hold for the count of three, release for three counts, then repeat three times. Do not press hard, just hold with a light pressure, but hard enough to feel the pressure. Now massage the kidney reflexes located on the head (Diagram 12). Remember, kidney problems can cause weak eyes.

When you do a complete body reflex workout, you will be stimulating the reflexes to the kidneys as well as the reflexes to the bladder and sex glands. See Photos 19, 42, 47, and 50 for methods of stimulating healing energy in the whole body.

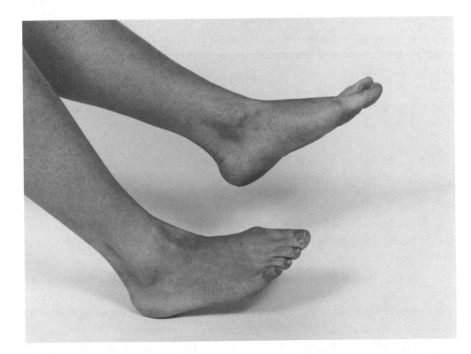

Photo 50: Pounding heels on the floor to stimulate circulation of energy throughout the body.

Faulty kidneys can lead to serious illnesses, so if you still have problems with your kidneys after a few days of reflex massage, you had better go to your naturopathic doctor. If a medical doctor is needed, he or she will advise you.

HELP FOR THE BLADDER

The main function of the bladder is to store urine for periodic release. It changes position and shape according to fullness. It is composed of a smooth muscle coat like that of the intestine but of greater thickness. Each kidney empties into a ureter, which then empties into the bladder. The bladder empties into the urethra, which conducts the urine from the bladder to the exterior.

On the inside of the foot, almost next to the pad of the heel, is a soft spongy area. See Diagram 5. You will find the reflexes in this area very tender if you are having any problems with the bladder. Using the thumb, massage any part that is tender with a gentle circular motion. Be sure to massage these reflexes on both feet. These reflexes are so near the location of the reflexes to the rectum, prostate, and lower spine that you will probably not be able to tell the difference as you massage the tenderness out. Remember, if it hurts, massage it out, because something in this area is not getting enough electrical life force to enable it to heal itself. You may also use heel pad massage to help the bladder. Just grab the heel pad in the hand and dig the fingers under it as shown in Photo 45. Always work the reflexes on both feet.

Using Hand and Foot Reflexes

Let us go to the hand reflexes for the bladder, in the web of the hand between the thumb and the forefinger. You will find reflexes to many parts of the body here, including the reflex to the bladder. If you find an "ouch" spot, either in the palm of the hand or on the back or top side, then massage it out.

Many types of bladder problems have been relieved by using these reflex techniques on the hands and the feet. These reflexes are very powerful in helping the body heal itself. See Diagrams 3 and 5.

As you massage the bladder reflexes on the feet, continue massaging on up the bottom of the foot to the center where the kidney reflex is located. Use this same technique as you massage the bladder reflexes in the hands. Massage from the soft area in front of the thumb on the palm of the hand and follow the reflexes to the ureters right up to the kidney reflexes in the center of the hand. Always do this massage to both hands and feet unless you are told differently. Now, let us pinch and massage the reflexes in the backs of the legs as we did the reflexes for hemorrhoids and prostate. No wonder these reflexes hurt so badly when massaged; they are related to so many parts of our lower extremities.

You will also massage the reflexes in the wrists, but instead of pinching cords, you will press and massage all areas of the wrist, searching out any tender buttons that you might find. This is to be done on the entire wrist, front and back. See Photo 38.

Using Head and Body Reflexes

When you follow the directions for stimulating the reflexes in the head, you will naturally be activating the reflexes to all these organs and glands. See Diagram 12 and Photos 10, 11, 12, and 51.

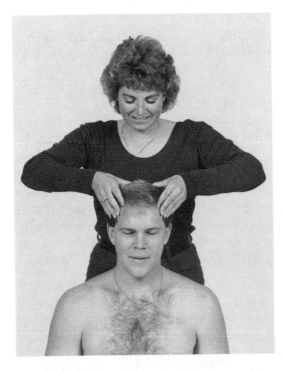

Photo 51: Position for massage of the reflexes in the head by another person.

Look at Diagrams 6, 7, and 8 to see where the bladder is located. Just above the pubic bone is a soft spongy area. Take the fingers of both hands and press in gently. You will be pressing on the bladder. Do not use a massaging motion here, but hold a steady pressure for a slow count of three, then release and count to three again. Do this three times. Now, place the palm of the right hand on this bladder area and place the palm of the left hand on top of the right hand and hold for a few moments. It will be best to do this on bare skin. If another person can do this for you, he or she will be sending an even stronger force of healing energy from the energy in his or her own body. This holds true for most of the reflex massages.

PROTEIN RELATED TO KIDNEY STONES

Too much protein in your diet can lead to kidney stones, a painful condition that afflicts an estimated one million Americans, according to a leading medical researcher.

Dr. Helen Linkswiler, a nutritionist at the University of Wisconsin, Madison, gave nine different combinations of purified protein and calcium supplements to fifteen male and female adult volunteers. She found that those volunteers who received high levels of protein lost calcium from their bodies even when they received calcium supplements. Lost calcium was excreted through the kidneys, where it could build up to form kidney stones, she explained.

Dr. Linkswiler has stated that her data show that high protein levels can be devastating to the bones. She believes that if we lost as much calcium as the volunteers did, sixty milligrams per day over a period of ten years, we would essentially have lost 10 to 25 percent of our body's calcium, 99 percent of which comes from our bones.

She added that those who received low levels of dietary protein did not lose calcium. People who took twenty-five grams of protein a day—about average for American adults—lost only a small amount.

Dr. Linkswiler advised that patients with kidneys stones be treated by reducing their protein intake rather than restricting calcium.

CHAPTER 17

Reflexology and the Sex Glands

The sex glands, or the glands of reproduction, are the easiest glands to regenerate back to health. No one knows the suffering that can be caused by the malfunctioning of these reproductive organs unless they have experienced such an ailment.

There have been too many unnecessary operations to remove these organs in women. In men, doctors operate to remove the prostate when natural methods of healing would have helped these organs return to health.

I have cured many men and women with the magic healing power of reflexology. Infertility, impotence, and prostate problems have been overcome by the simple method of pressing and massaging certain reflex buttons. I have received many letters telling me of several cases in which reflexology helped to overcome impotence.

How Reflexology Overcame a Man's Impotence

Dear Mildred Carter,

I had been giving reflexology treatments to an elderly couple for some time when they said they wanted to talk to me about a personal matter. It was embarrassing for them to tell me that the man was completely impotent. They wanted to know if reflexology could help. I assured them that it could and went to work on reflexes to stimulate the man's gonads (sex glands).

I was a little surprised when they told me on their next visit that the treatment had worked and they were as happy as newly-weds. The wife had tears in her eyes as she thanked me and said they had always had a happy life together until he became impotent. Now their happiness was complete once more.

—A Student

Reflexology Awakens Woman's Sexual Desire After Forty Years

Dear Mrs. Carter,

I have been married for forty miserable years. I have a wonderful wife, whom I have always loved with all of my heart, but she was not interested in sex all of those years. I thought she hated me! I got so I didn't bother to touch her or even kiss her anymore. Then, after talking to you on the phone about reflexology, and then reading your wonderful letter, we decided to try your method. God, did it work. For the first time in our marriage, we feel like newlyweds. We are so grateful to you, and we hope you will help many others like us who have been living in the darkness of ignorance.

—M.B. & K.B.

SEX IS IMPORTANT TO GOOD HEALTH

We all know that a normal sex life is important to good health. If our organs of reproduction are diseased and malfunctioning, or if we are having psychological or emotional problems, we cannot enjoy normal, satisfactory sexual experiences.

Sex is one of the strongest drives in the animal world, and in humans it has a more important function than to create new life. When the sex urge begins to diminish, it is a sure sign of the slowing down of one or more of the endocrine glands that are directly responsible for the overall health and well-being of the body. Reflexology can stimulate the endocrine glands, increase your sex drive and your hormone production, and retard the process of aging. One eighty-six-year-old woman told me that she thinks reflexology is "real sexy."

BODY REFLEXES TO STIMULATE SEX GLANDS FOR MEN AND WOMEN

Look at Diagram 12 and find the reflexes to the sex organs on the head and also the other endocrine glands (pituitary, pineal, thyroid, parathyroid, thymus, pancreas, and adrenals). All these reflexes will stimulate the organs and glands named when pressed, massaged, or tapped. Light tapping with the fists or with the wire brush and also massaging with the fingers will bring renewed circulations. See Photos 10, 11 and 16.

First, we will turn to the reflexes in the pituitary glands, the thyroid, and the adrenals, which have a large influence on the gonads in both male and female. It has been scientifically proven that one of the main causes of disorder in the reproductive organs is an imbalance of hormones. By massaging the reflexes to these special endocrine glands, you are stimulating them to produce the hormones that are needed to normalize the gonads. See Diagram 2 of the hand and feet. Study the directions in the endocrine chapter for massaging the reflexes on the hands and the feet to open up channels that will send energy and a renewed flow of hormones into all areas of the gonads. This will bring them into healthy, normal harmony and balance with the whole system.

In Diagrams 7 and 8, notice the reflex buttons near the internal organs and glands. With the middle finger, or all the fingers grouped together, press into each one of these reflexes that are in relation to the sex glands, and also the reflexes that correspond with the endocrine glands. Press each reflex and count to three slowly, then release. Repeat until you have pressed each one five times. If there is a lot of fat involved, you will have to press in deeply to reach the reflex button. Do this gently so as not to bruise the flesh. Also press the reflex button to the solar plexus. See Photo 4 and press about one inch higher than is shown for solar plexus reflex.

The Medulla Oblongata

Now let us go to that vitality-generating reflex button, the medulla oblongata, which is called the power station of life forces. In Diagram

13 you will see the location of this all-important reflex button. When pressure is applied here, it prepares the body for sustained action; the impulses are funneled into it from your entire nerve network. It steps up vitality and relieves tensions, so you can easily understand why it is called a giant power station and will help in stimulating the sex glands.

With the middle finger of both hands, or just one finger, press this reflex button and hold to the count of three. Do this about five times to make sure all the other glands are getting an equal flow of the life force.

ALTERNATING PRESSURE ON THE ARMS AND LEGS

There are several reflex buttons that stimulate the sex glands on the arms and the legs, but rather than confuse you with too many reflexes to remember, I suggest that you use the reflex roller as illustrated in Photo 41. This will help you locate any hidden reflex buttons that may indicate blockages that you would not be aware of otherwise. Do not use this method on legs if you have varicose veins.

Roll the roller massager on the inside of the leg, starting at the ankle. Roll it up along the calf of the leg to the knee. You may want to roll this same area several times. Then, move the roller toward the front bone and roll up and down again. You will be amazed at the "ouch" spots you will find. It is no wonder that you have been having so many health problems! Remember, the blockage you are releasing here is not only going to the sex glands but to nearly every part of your body. Now, roll up and down on the outside of the leg. If you prefer to massage each tender button as you discover it with the roller, you may use the fingers to massage it out. I like to use the roller because it does work wonders in contacting a lot of blocked channels that would otherwise go untreated. It also stimulates the flow of the lymph fluid. Use the roller to search out any "ouch" buttons that might be in the calf of the leg. Don't neglect rolling it around the knees in various places. Be sure to do this to both legs.

Move to the upper legs, the thighs. Ah, here is where you will cry uncle! You will probably find so many very sore buttons that you won't believe it possible to have that many sore spots and not be aware of it. Starting at the knee on the inside of the leg, roll the reflex roller all the way up to the crotch. Continue rolling the whole leg.

When you get to the outside of the leg, roll up onto the hip. You will probably find some "ouch" buttons here, also.

Remember, you do not have to press very hard to get results. In most cases, it does not take much pressure to loosen the obstructions and open the channels.

Now let us go to the arms and give them the same rolling reflexology treatment that you used on the legs. I like to use the same roller massager on other parts of the body too, as it seems to search out congested reflexes that I miss when using only my fingers and it does it in a much shorter time.

THE BACK

The back is also involved in stimulating the sex glands, but it is impossible to massage the full length of the back by yourself, so let us hope you can find someone to roll the massager on each side of your spine. *Do not use the roller directly on the spine.* You can probably reach the lower part of each side of the spine by yourself with the roller massager. Do the best that you can if you have no one to help you. See Diagram 6B. Also massage the reflexes marked on the buttocks.

Another way to help stimulate the gonads is to massage the lower back muscles. Use the fingers here as you massage across the muscles from the spine to the hips with a rolling massaging motion.

USING REFLEX TONGUE PROBE

Another excellent way to stimulate the gonads is with the reflex tongue probe. This is a magic little massager that you can use to reach the reflexes to the gonads located on the tongue. See Photo 22. We have many stories of the wonderful results people are getting from using the tongue probe. Look at Diagram 16 (page 54) on zone therapy and notice how the center lines run through the tongue and straight down through the gonads (uterus and penis). Now you understand why the reflexes in the tongue are sure to send the life force into the sex glands.

OVERCOMING IMPOTENCE

For added stimulation for those who feel they need still further help to overcome impotence, take the scrotum and its contents (testicles) in the hand and apply on and off pressure about twenty times (or more) a day. Let us look at a so-called "hot spot" which is located between the scrotum and the anus and another key stimulation button that is located between the tail bone (coccyx) and the anus. Press and release these sex-stimulating reflex buttons with the fingers, gently, five times. Now, for further stimulation, press all around the anus. Massaging these sex-stimulating reflexes can be useful for women as well as men.

An Example from the Philippines

While I was in the Philippines, I met a lady who was going to the same healer I was. She told me that her husband was impotent, but she was too embarrassed to ask if there was a way to help him. Since this healer and I were good friends and he was teaching me his ways of natural healing, I was not shy in broaching the subject with him. Using her as a patient, he showed me how to bring the blood to the area that would stimulate the sex organ. It was quite painful to her and she screamed and yelled, but he kept right on showing me what to do and telling her to listen and learn the technique.

He had her spread her legs while lying down and, placing his fingers on the inside of both legs near the rectum, he searched for the tender spots. He showed me how the vein crossed over the bony structure and was quite tender. Now, he kept pressure on this vein and pulled the blood up toward the clitoris (the penis on men). He said the blood slows down in this protected area and all it needs is to be pulled up a few times to start the renewal of circulation, which will end all symptoms of impotency. He also pressed the blood down the inside of the leg to the heel.

This is easy to understand and also to practice. Because many of us get very little exercise, it is easy to understand that the circulation of the blood is slowed down over the years. So, if you are having sex problems, this would probably be one of the main areas to work on.

Your Voice Affects Your Virility

I will give you a million-dollar secret from the Himalayan monasteries:
At a meeting, we learned that when a man's voice begins to become high-pitched, it is a sure sign that his virility is in a deplorable condition. The vortex at the base of the neck controls the vocal cords

and is directly connected with the vortex below, in the sex center. What affects one affects the other. When a man's voice is high, his manly vitality is low.

You can increase the speed of vibration in these vortexes by lowering the voice. Listen to the deep voice of a virile man, and make yourself speak in a deep masculine voice as much as possible. Some of you may find this hard to do, but it will bring results. Your lowered voice will speed up the vortex in the sex center, which will improve your masculine energy.

REFLEXOLOGY TO BUILD HEALTHY SEX ORGANS IN THE MALE

The most important glands to stimulate for healthy functioning of the gonads (sex gland) are the endocrine glands. Make sure that you massage the reflexes to these glands first, as explained in the chapter on endocrine glands. If any of these reflexes are tender, they may contribute to trouble with the sex glands. If you have ever suffered from a malfunction of the sex glands, you already know that it hurts from the waist down.

Let us look to the reflexes related to the penis and the testicles. There are many reflexes to these, but I have had such wonderful results with a few simple ones that I will not confuse you with many.

Press in on the sex reflex button about the width of the hand below the navel, either with the thumb or the fingers, and massage the area rather hard for a slow count of three. See Diagram 7.

On the inside of the leg, about one hand's width above the ankle (Diagrams 6C and 6F), is a reflex to the gonads. It will probably be very tender if you have any malfunctioning of the sex organs. Massage this reflex with the thumb, gently at first, until you work out some of the soreness. This might take several days. Do not massage too long at first, not over thirty seconds. The whole area may be sore, so take time and massage all the area near this "ouch" button. See Photo 52 and Diagrams 6C and 6F.

About three inches above the knee, on the soft area on the outside of the knee, is another very tender reflex. It will make itself known quickly if your sex glands are malfunctioning. See Diagram 6C. Use the same massage on this as you did lower on the leg.

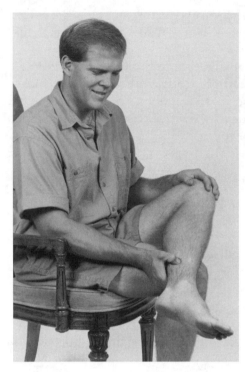

Photo 52: Position for pressing reflex buttons to overcome impotency.

Let us turn to a reflex on the back. You may have to have someone else help with this. If you try it yourself, place your hands on your hips with the fingers pointing toward the abdomen. Now, slide the hands toward the back. Just before you reach the spine, press in and find the tender reflex buttons. This will be in the vicinity of the lumbar disc. See Diagram 6B. Notice also the reflexes marked on the buttocks. Press these with one finger and hold for quick stimulation. These back reflex buttons are especially helpful to those who have problems with erection.

Now look below the ankles. Notice on Diagram 4 where the reflexes are located to stimulate the testicles and the penis.

Reflex Buttons on the Heels

The next reflex area involves the heels. Yes, I mean the *whole heel*. You will not believe the pain that can be invoked by pressing the reflexes around the whole pad of the heel on both feet if you have any malfunctioning of the sex glands or colon or any part of the lower extremities. You will probably need one of the reflex devices, such as the hand probe or the comb, to get good results in this area. It may take several treatments to work out all the tenderness. It is important that you do keep massaging the tender buttons until they are no longer sore, but not in one day.

Start with the fingers hooked under the pad of the heel near the center of the foot and press in with a massaging motion. See Photo 45. After a few seconds, move the fingers slowly around the heel pad. I am talking about the heel *pad*, not the bony part where the reflexes to the hemorrhoids are located. By looking at Diagram 5 you will see that the reflexes to the small intestines are also located near this area. So if you want to rejuvenate your sex glands, you can see why you will have to clear up other problems of the lower area of the body.

How to Give Yourself a Testicular Exam

I have received many letters from men asking how to check themselves for testicular cancer. It is very easy for most men to perform this simple testicular exam on themselves; it takes only a minute or two, and should be done every month. You can examine yourself while in the shower, while the skin of the scrotum is relaxed, and the testes are easy to feel.

Examine one testicle at a time, and be very gentle, so as not to hurt yourself. Using both hands, place your index and middle fingers underneath one of your testes. Now place your thumbs on top. Gently rolling it, you will feel a somewhat firm, oval, testis. It should be smooth and free of lumps. You will feel the epididymis, on the back side of each testicle; this is the sperm storage duct, and will feel a little spongier. Search for suspicious, hard lumps or swollen areas on the testicle.

Use reflexology to maintain the health of your reproductive organs, concentrating on the gonad reflexes and all the other endocrine glands. The male reproductive system is very sensitive, so when reflexing this area start out slowly and use a gentle touch.

Operation Avoided for a Baby

One of my reflexology students told me of her experience with her grandson. When the baby was born there was something wrong with his scrotum. The doctors said he needed to have an operation, but they would have to wait a few weeks to perform it because he was too young to survive it.

Mrs. M.'s children did not believe in reflexology and made fun of her for practicing it. One night they asked her if she would keep the baby overnight, because they had to make a business trip and would rather not take him along with them.

After they were gone the baby cried a lot, so Mrs. M. took his little feet in her hands and started applying basic reflexology to the reflexes on the bottom of them.

When she touched one particular place, he would jerk his little foot as if it were hurting him. So every hour or so she went back and massaged the reflexes in his feet very carefully and gently for only a few seconds at a time. She did this several times while the baby was with her. The next morning when he took his bottle, he seemed to be taking milk normally and didn't cry anymore.

The mother and father picked the baby up and took him home. Nothing was said about his condition. Later in the day the daughter called her mother and said, "Mother, you didn't."

The mother said, "Yes, I did."

They both knew what they were talking about. She said, "I should tell you, my baby is well. The problem has completely vanished." And it was true. The baby was well and the operation was never performed.

HOW TO HELP PROSTATE TROUBLE

Nearly all of the cases of prostate trouble that I have ever worked on with reflexology have been helped. If massaging the reflexes to the penis does not bring you relief from prostate trouble after several days, you might try Mrs. Therese Pfrimmer's method. See if there is a hard band around the base of the penis. If you find that this is so, try massaging this band with the fingers until it becomes pliable and eventually vanishes. Your physician should be able to tell you if there is any sign of a more serious problem before you go into this deep massage of the penis.

Prostate Problems Cured

Dear Mrs. Carter,

I am a working reflexologist and now have many satisfied patients. In fact one of my patients had an appointment to have a gland operation, but I told him to hold off for at least four treatments on his feet. He followed my advice. He called me about a week after the fourth treatment and said the swelling went down to normal on his prostate glands and that an operation was not necessary. The patient then wrote me a letter thanking me for the treatments. There have been many other patients with gallstones, back trouble, sinus problems, hemorrhoids, and many other disorders that have been healed by reflexology. When I can help people regain their health it makes me feel good also.

Thanking you kindly,

—Mr. K.O.B.

Dear Ms. Carter,

I am a man of seventy-four years. I have one of your books on hand reflexology and I have had good results from different aches and pains.

A few months ago, I had trouble with my prostate gland. My doctor said I would have to have surgery, but I followed your instructions and now my prostate is fine again. I really believe in reflexology and use this book all the time. Thank you.

—Mr. R.A.R.

Reflexology to Prostate Helps Man Sleep

Dear Mrs. Carter,

I am seventy-five years old, and for years I have had a developing problem with Nocturia, and had to get up five times to use the bathroom because of prostate problems. After trying reflexology on my prostate, I slept from 1:30 A.M. until 7:30 A.M. the first night, which I hadn't done for years, and I also slept unbroken, wonderfully restful sleep from midnight until 8:15 A.M. the next night; I hadn't done that since my youth.

I am most grateful.

Sincerely yours,

—L.G.

How to Subdue Sexual Energy

For those who are not sexually active, here is a special exercise to keep the sex urge subdued.

First, relax completely for a few minutes; then sit up straight. Keeping the neck and head very relaxed, start breathing deeply. Take five or six breaths, close your eyes, and try to visualize a great force within you. Try not to have any thoughts connected with sex at this time. Resume the deep breathing, and each time you inhale, imagine that you draw the sexual energy upward from its center, the base of the spine. Each time you exhale, direct this force to the solar plexus or, if you prefer, to the brain, to be stored there. Keep on doing this exercise for a few minutes without interrupting the rhythm of your breath. If you are not used to doing these deep-breathing exercises, stop them if you begin to feel dizzy. You may resume them after three or four hours, if necessary. You must be able to will strongly that the sexual energies rise upward before being directed to the solar plexus or the head.

An Exercise for Bladder Control

Here is a good exercise for women who have weak bladder control. It will strengthen the muscles of the lower extremities and also weak abdominal muscles.

When you sit on the toilet to urinate, squeeze the muscle shut to stop the flow of urine—hold—then release. Repeat as often as possible, at least ten times. When you pull the muscles together to stop the urine, also pull in on the muscles of the abdomen. You will be tightening and strengthening important body muscles pertaining to the gonads and a better sex life.

For additional bladder control, after you urinate, lean forward slightly and try again to urinate to make sure you have drained all fluids from the bladder. Sometimes it helps to stand up after urinating, then sit back down and try again. By making sure the bladder is empty, you may not have to make so many trips to the bathroom.

Mrs. K.'s Problem

Mrs. K. tells us of her experiences of not being able to hold her urine. She was a young mother and it got so bad she didn't dare leave the house. Her chiropractor told her to strengthen the muscles by doing the exercise just described. She did and has never had that problem since. She is now a grandmother.

USING REFLEX TONGUE PROBE TO RELIEVE CRAMPS

I want to tell you of the importance of the reflex tongue probe in helping relieve complaints of the gonads, especially in relieving cramps. You can see in Diagram 16 on page 54 that line 1 runs down through the center of the body to the uterus. When you put pressure on the tongue by using the reflex tongue probe, you stimulate all areas along zone 1. See Photo 22. You will probably find some very tender reflexes here, especially near your period time. Many women carry a tongue probe in their purse at all times to help alleviate the pain of unexpected cramps and other symptoms of discomfort that might arise. Don't forget the value of the reflex comb. See the chapter on reflex devices.

This was used by medical doctors not too many years ago to alleviate all types of ailments, including headaches, earaches, backaches, and even to aid in painless childbirth.

HOW TO USE REFLEXOLOGY FOR PAINLESS CHILDBIRTH

This chapter would not be complete if I didn't tell you of a simple, natural method of painless childbirth. Reflexology is a boon to expectant mothers who choose to have their babies at home; they welcome this natural, painless method of delivery with no drugs or anesthetics to endanger their health and the lives of their unborn infants.

Do not use this technique before the baby is ready to be born. It might cause it to be born too soon and lessen its chances for survival.

The truly natural method of delivering a child is not to lie down but to stand on the feet and squat. This was the natural way native women had babies for hundreds of years. Some women still use their natural instincts to deliver in this method when they are not strapped down to a delivery table in a hospital.

With the help of two combs, a woman starting into delivery can press the teeth of the combs into the reflexes of her hands to help relax the muscles, allowing the baby to be born in a short time with very little pain. This makes the birth easier for the mother and the baby, reducing the likelihood of complications.

As soon as labor pains begin, the mother should be given a comb for each hand and something solid to press her feet against. Although ordinary household combs can be used, they are apt to break under pressure and injure the fingers. For this reason, reflex combs, which are specially designed for the purposes of hand reflexology, are recommended.

Holding the combs' teeth down, the patient exerts pressure across the tops by pressing down firmly with the fingers until the teeth dig into the palm area, as hard as can be comfortably borne and maintaining constant pressure. If the hands become tired, relax them for a few minutes; then continue the pressure. The combs should be held across the palm, or wherever it seems most comfortable to the patient. At the same time press the soles of the feet hard against a footboard, which should have a rough rather than a smooth surface.

The patient might find more relief by turning the combs upside down and pressing the teeth into the tips of the fingers and the ends of the thumbs. See Photo 21.

Women in Labor Instinctively Use Reflexology Technique

This method of pressure on the hands has always been used by women in labor. It is a natural instinct to clench the hands or grasp the hands of anyone near. This is nature's own method of bringing relief from pain in labor. This is inadequate, however, because the pressure is not maintained for a sufficient length of time and because the means of the pressure is not sufficiently "sharp." Reflexology increases the effectiveness of an already existing method by improving on it.

Labor Pains Relieved by Reflexology

Reflexology relieves the nagging pains in the first stage of labor, not by retarding, but rather by promoting dilation. In the second stage, delivery is hastened and the mother delivers quickly and painlessly. Dr. White tells us that when using this method of helping the mother to a painless and quick delivery, there is absolutely no danger to either the mother or the child. By using reflexology, you need no longer resort to harmful drugs to alleviate the pain and discomfort of childbirth.

How Reflexology Saved an Unborn Baby

My daughter tried for several years to have a baby, with no success. When she did finally become pregnant, her doctor was not aware of it and operated on the uterus. She lost that baby at four months, and her doctor warned her that she could never carry a baby, and if she did, it would have all kinds of defects. That really frightened her and her husband.

I told her that he was not telling the truth, so she changed doctors after she became pregnant again. When she was in her fourth month, the baby stopped moving! The stories the first doctor had told her came to mind, and she thought she would lose this baby, too. A friend's mother was a masseuse, so she went to her for help. The woman massaged and pressed on every reflex she knew, without results. Then she told her there was one last chance, and she pressed on a certain reflex button on top of my daughter's head. The baby gave a big kick and started moving around. They both cried with joy.

You can see that perfectly healthy baby girl in some of the pictures in this book.

Look at Diagram 12 for the reflexes on top of the head that go to the sex glands (gonads) and also those for the adrenal glands. The adrenal reflexes are probably what sparked renewed life and energy into the unborn baby. The body warmer reflexes, located along the top of the head, probably also helped by stimulating a weakening flame of life force. See Diagram 14.

A WONDERFUL TONIC

I cannot end this chapter without mentioning the wonderful help women of all ages get from the tonic "Lydia Pinkham"—a mixture of special herbs. I gave it to my daughters as soon as they started to develop into womanhood and I still have a bottle of Lydia Pinkham on my shelf. I wouldn't think of being without it. I usually have to order it ahead, as it is becoming hard to get and some drugstores won't bother to order it. If I feel the least bit of stress in the area of my lower abdomen, I start taking the tonic—all symptoms of discomfort vanish within a day. You see, it relaxes the reproductive organs that tend to tighten up under stress. It accomplishes from the inside what reflexology does from the outside. The two methods combine and help bring the miracle of harmony and relaxation back to the whole reproductive system.

I had a young girl come to me for treatment because she couldn't get pregnant. I treated her for a few times and told her about the Lydia Pinkham tonic. In a very short time, she informed me that she was pregnant and she later gave birth to a perfect baby girl.

Lydia Pinkham is the best tonic I know of to carry one through the menopause. This may be of benefit to men also, when they reach the change-of-life age, in relaxing their gonads. I never knew when I went through the menopause because one month it was there and then it was gone forever, with no adverse effects. If you can no longer get Lydia Pinkham, then try your health food store for special mixed herbs to take its place.

CHAPTER 18

How Reflexology Helps Premenstrual Syndrome and Menopause

To help you relax and feel more comfortable you will want the healing power of nature to open up pathways that will revitalize your system and give renewed strength to your bodily processes. You can prevent PMS and the discomforts of menopause with the healing energy of reflexology, as it tones up your system and brings well-being to your body.

REFLEXOLOGY AND PMS

Before menstruation starts, there are several techniques you can use to help stop the pain and discomfort brought on by hormonal imbalances. First, it is always best to give yourself a complete reflexology workout to activate the healing powers in your body and help balance the whole system. Give yourself a complete reflex workout at least twice a week, beginning two weeks before your menstrual cycle begins. This is when hormonal changes start to take place within your body. These changes influence the rise of salt and fluids in your system, and you may notice a puffy feeling. Reflexology stimulates circulation to wash away retained fluids and relieve the heaviness and bloated feeling. It is wise to cut back on salty foods such as chips, nuts, and crackers. I find by adding a salt enhancer to my foods, such as lemon juice, it perks up the flavor without causing fluid buildup in my body.

Now I want you to make yourself comfortable, get into a relaxed position so that you can easily work on one of your feet. You will want to send healing energy up through your foot, along the internal pathway, up to your pelvic area. Take hold of your right foot, place two fingers, or your thumb, in the fleshy part on the outside of the foot, between the ankle bone and the heel. With the press-and-roll technique, work this area completely, all around the ankle on the outer side of the foot. This is the reflex to the ovaries, massaging clear over to the back of the ankle and working down underneath it, searching for specific tender spots. It might be more convenient for you to use the thumb for this particular reflex. Now move back to the left foot, using the same procedure, working about the ankle on the outside of the left foot. If you are having trouble with the ovaries this area will be extremely painful; you can use a light touch here.

Now let us move to the inside of the foot, and work the reflex to the uterus with the thumb or finger. Press into the soft area just under the ankle bone. Massage all around the ankle on the inside of the foot. You may find that the reflex will be very sore under the ankle bone and back a little toward the heel. Remember to be very gentle when the reflex is extremely tender. Do not overmassage; just a short workout the first few times can do much more good than massaging too much. Now change feet to give the reflexes on the right foot a rest, while you work the reflexes to these same glands on the inside and outside of the left foot. Now using your thumb and finger you will gently press into the depressions behind the ankles, and back toward your heel. Now press along the sides of your Achilles tendon, moving on up toward your calf muscle. Use a press-and-pinch method here.

Now you will want to work the rest of the foot, using a gentle, deep pressure, massaging systematically up the foot. Start with your toes and work to the heel. Press hard enough to reach the inner reflex points beneath the skin. Give yourself a complete reflex workout, rubbing every button to balance your whole system.

As you work on up and over the reflexes, you may find a very painful spot. If this happens, work the reflex briefly, then go on to another reflex. You can return to the very painful spot later. After you work other areas, come back to the very painful spot and work it again. Remember never to overwork a reflex as you can bruise the sensitive areas. Eventually you will work the pain out. Although it may take several sessions, as the pain eases, it means the blood is flowing freely again, flushing out all sluggishness and poisons. You will soon experience the vitalizing, pain-free health you deserve.

HOW REFLEXOLOGY HELPS OVERCOME MOOD SWINGS AND DEPRESSION

Remember the importance of your endocrine glands when you are massaging your reflexes. You will want to keep this entire system healthy, as this major system is a powerful coordinator of all body functions. These glands strengthen and regulate body rhythms, as well as balance chemical and emotional functions which will have a direct affect on your mood. Study Diagram 2, and give *all* these glands some additional attention.

We know how important it is for a woman's system to be in complete harmony to avoid mood swings. The thyroid is a reflex button that we will use to bring on a good mood. When the thyroid gland is not functioning properly, our body may start to feel "down" or depressed. Tests have shown that when the function of the thyroid is decreased, the function of the brain is also decreased by the same amount, thus resulting in depression or negative emotions. You will find the reflex button to the thyroid on your hands, feet or neck. See Photos 27, 28, 29, and 30.

In addition to the endocrine glands, lightly work the reflexes to the liver, lungs, solar plexus, and brain. Whenever you are feeling stressed, you will want to massage these vital reflexes to help overcome depression. (Remember, the liver is a sensitive reflex, so you will not want to overmassage it.) Work the whole liver reflex area for about seven seconds. A sluggish liver can affect menstrual pain, cause stress, and upset your whole system. However, when the liver is functioning properly it performs many tasks, such as cleaning the blood and distributing needed vitamins and minerals throughout the body. (See Chapter 14 for more information on the liver.)

Your whole system benefits from reflexology. With its use many women notice they become much more relaxed before and during their menstrual cycle. Use additional health-building methods such as body movement to limber up. You can take long brisk walks, and breathe deeply, to get your circulation stimulated, this will also help alleviate depression. Soon you will feel a great improvement in your health and disposition. As you relieve body stiffness, you will also be relieving mental rigidity. Both your appearance and behavior will improve as your body returns to health.

REFLEX THE URINARY SYSTEM

You will want to keep the kidneys, bladder, and urethra strong and healthy. Remember to drink eight glasses of fresh, natural water every day. Your kidneys control and balance the chemicals and water in your blood. They work hard to filter wastes and maintain proper fluid balance. Work the reflexes to the kidneys and bladder. Now massage between these two areas, as you work back and forth you will also be stimulating the ureter reflex.

Keep your kidneys healthy by working the reflex points on your hands and feet. They lie lengthwise, just below the adrenal reflex, almost in the center of each foot, and in each hand. See Diagrams 3 and 5.

You can also rub and massage over the kidneys by placing both your hands on your hips, fingers facing to the back of your body, thumbs to the front. Now place fingers of both hands just above your waistline on back and work the kidney areas with a pressing, circular movement. Continue on down to the lower end of the tailbone. Repeat twice. Soon all tensions disappear as nature works freely, relieving pain, as fluids move away from congested organs.

HOW TO RELAX AND RELIEVE CRAMPS

One way to relieve cramps and tension in the ovaries is to rock your pelvis by either lying on your back or sitting up and bending your knees, placing both feet flat on the floor. Sway your knees to the left, then to the right about eight inches in each direction.

I learned another technique many years ago when my youngest daughter started her period at school. She felt a little dizzy and had very bad cramps, so she went to the school nurse's office to lie down. This nurse was wonderful; instead of giving my daughter a pill for the pain, she explained a bit of anatomy, telling her that the stomach is mostly on the left side of our body, and when we lie on the left side, it takes the pressure off the uterus and the cramps stop. This worked wonders; it took away the pain and was also very comforting. My daughter now uses this same technique with her own teenage daughter.

I received a letter from Mrs. R. who wrote that she was helped immensely with the use of reflexology.

Dear Mrs. Carter,

I have always had bad menstrual cramps. My husband and I build houses, and the hard work and heavy lifting made them even worse. It got so that I had to stay home for two days every month. I honestly could hardly walk standing straight. Since I have been working on the reflexes, this has greatly improved. Sometimes I don't notice the cramps at all. Also my hair was always thin and would never grow past my shoulders no matter what I did. Working the reflexes on my scalp and rubbing my fingernails together has my hair thicker and it is now just past my waist! I really like your technique of face-lift, it works wonders for wrinkles! I would never have believed anything like this to be true.

—Mrs. D.R., Canada

A Natural Sedative

If body tensions or cramps are keeping you awake, try this effective, relaxing sleep therapy.

Lying on your back, in a quiet place, allow your body to go limp. Close your eyes and breathe slowly and deeply. Practice deep breathing four or five times until you feel a warm calmness come over you. Now concentrate on relaxing *all* tensions; mentally visualize each part of your body and relax each of them, one at a time.

First inhale a deep breath, now tighten the muscles in your toes, ankles, and feet. Hold for seven seconds, then exhale and relax. Again...breathe in slowly, this time tighten your toes, ankles, feet, calves, and kneecaps, hold for seven seconds, exhale, and relax....Slowly continue this routine until you have included all the muscles, tissues, and organs from the tip of your toes to the top of your head. Finally, tightening your entire body, even your chin, and every part of your face including your throat, tongue, and mouth, close your eyes very tightly, and wrinkle your nose. Now you should have your whole body in a very tight, stiff and tense position. . . . . Exhale and relax.

Now that you are completely relaxed, place your left hand just below your navel and press for a sedating, soothing, and cleaning effect. If this area is tender, work it in a slow, gentle, circular motion for seven seconds, and then take a slow deep breath. Repeat several times. Now your body is totally relaxed on the inside, as well as the outside, your cramps have stopped and you can benefit from a fully relaxed and restful sleep.

How to Stop Pain

The pain of cramps or headaches may start when you are busy at work. If this happens you may not have time for a complete reflex workout. However, you can turn to your hands for pain relief. Work the reflex points to the reproductive and circulatory systems, and then spend a few minutes on the endocrine gland reflexes; as you have learned, they coordinate all your body functions.

Nature has provided a very convenient place on your hand for a special reflex point that will relieve pain in many parts of the body. This point is especially helpful when one is suffering with cramps. To find this point, make a fist, and you will notice a small mound where the thumb and index finger meet. The reflex button is beneath the peak of this mound. Work this point to trigger the release of natural cortisone, which will help diminish your cramps. See Photos 35 and "C."

Work this point, and the reflexes all around your thumb to relieve your headache.

HOW REFLEXOLOGY HELPS SORE BREASTS

If there is pain or tenderness in the breast it may be from an imbalance of estrogen or progesterone. A complete reflex workout to all reflexes on your feet, hands, or specific areas of your head, will help improve circulation to reduce swelling and pain. Be persistent and faithful in working the reflex points to the breast, which you will find on the top of each foot and hand. See Diagram 4.

Also, you will want to work the reflexes to the endocrine glands, lungs, and lymph system. To work the lymph glands, you will press across the top of each foot or on each wrist using your fingers, thumb or heel of your hand. See Photo G. You may want to rotate your ankles in one direction, stop, and rotate in the other direction...or pump your lymph glands. To do this you will want to lay on your back, with legs elevated, point toes up and then down, for one or two minutes; also from side to side. Also pump lymph nodes at wrist. This action will help to clear away blocked or infected lymph fluid.

Many physical conditions related to hormonal changes have been greatly helped by using pressure on the tongue. You may notice an odd tingling sensation in quite another part of your body, and you will know that the connection of healing energy is getting through. See Chapter 5, How to Use Reflex Massage on the Tongue.

Castor Oil Packs for Sore Breasts

Breast inflammation and minor infections may be gone in no time with this secret from Gaylord Hauser. I have used this special technique to get rid of pain and inflammation for many years. It can be used anywhere on the body to draw out infections. Cold-pressed castor oil contains a substance that increases T11 lymphocyte function, which will speed the healing of all infections, and take away the pain. I always keep my castor oil and used wool flannel cloth sealed in a freezer-strong zip lock bag in the refrigerator.

You will need cold-pressed castor oil, a wool flannel cloth, a piece of plastic, and your heating pad. Fold the flannel cloth several times and put a lot of castor oil on it, enough to saturate the cloth, but not so much that it will run off or drip onto the breast. Place the cloth onto the breast, then apply the plastic over the cloth, now place the heating pad on top. Turn it to a hot setting; if this is uncomfortable, turn it down to the medium setting. Leave it on for at least one hour. Use this castor oil pack as needed, once a day for three to seven days, and it will draw out congestion. It can be used more frequently without any harmful effects. After one week you should be free of all inflammation.

Castor oil packs are wonderful for drawing out all kinds of congestion and have helped many illnesses just disappear. I have used this combination of reflex therapy and castor oil packs for many years, and it always proves to be a true blessing. I received a call from a young man who described his wife as being very ill. He said, "She seems to have everything wrong with her!" This couple had been married just over one year, and Dan was very worried about his wife. He told me that she felt so ill she had not wanted to get out of bed for almost a month. The doctors found nothing wrong with her after taking several blood tests. They suggested further testing.

Dan had been taking time off from work to care for his wife. By this time he was desperate for help but did not want the doctors to run more tests. I told him we could help her naturally with reflexology and castor oil packs. He was determined to help his wife return to health. She also agreed to help herself in any way she could. So we started our work.

First, I gave her a complete foot reflexology workout, sending energy to all her organs and glands. I worked slowly for thirty minutes on each foot, making sure not to miss any of her endocrine glands, and gave her lymph reflexes extra attention.

We then used the castor oil pack method I just described and placed the pack on her stomach and chest. We left the pack on for two hours, then turned her over and placed the pack on her back for two hours. She complained of pains in her legs, so we placed the pack on her legs for two hours. She then told us that she felt a great deal of congestion in her chest, so we started over with the castor oil pack on her chest for two hours. After this she felt better, and drank a cup of garlic soup.

Four hours later we repeated the procedure, this time placing the pack on each area for only one hour at a time.

For the next two days, Dan would alternate the castor oil packs every one or two hours, and at the same time, he would work a few of the reflexes on her hands for about ten minutes, making sure to rub the reflex to the lymph glands. He worked across the back of her wrist several times to help nature release any congestion that might be invading his wife's body. Once a day he would give her a complete foot reflexology workout.

Dan was rewarded for the many hours he spent helping his wife return to health. His love and devotion paid off. After only two days, his wife's appetite improved, and soon she was able to sit up, then walk. As she began to feel better, she worked the reflexes on her own hands, and continued to use the oil pack twice a day (to the stomach and back), and within two weeks she was well and strong enough to return to her job.

I kept in close contact with Dan, and soon he reported the good news that his wife was feeling great. She was strong and healthy again, with no pain or congestion of any kind. In fact she had joined a softball team and was playing tennis. After receiving a good check-up from her doctor, their future plans include a healthy diet, weekly reflex treatments, and maybe with a little luck plans to have a baby.

Cool Your Breasts

You will find relief from hot swollen breasts by using a gentle, cool rub. Place your hands under cold running water, or in a bowl of cool water; slightly shake most of the water from your hands, and then cup them over the breasts. While hands are in this position gently massage to ease the fluids back into the lymph passages. This will feel very refreshing and also help promote healing. Repeat several times.

MENOPAUSE, A NEW BEGINNING

As a woman's body adjusts to the hormonal changes of menopause, it often causes mood swings, hot flashes, and insomnia. You do not have to experience any of these symptoms if you take Lydia Pinkham Liquid. It soothes the agony of hot flashes and discomfort suffered at the time of menopause. Always check with your doctor when using any home remedy if your symptoms persist.

You will want to work the reflex points to your endocrine system to regulate and balance blood sugars. Also massage the reflexes to your brain and spine, which you will find on either your hands or feet. See Diagrams 3 and 5. Feel the bony instep on the inside edge of your foot (or down index finger on hand). As your spine relaxes, so will you. Your whole body receives its nerve supply from your brain and spine. The nerves branch out at intervals from the vertebral column and penetrate all parts of your body. The reflexes to the spine or other bone areas may be worked for an unlimited time, unlike reflexes to glands and organs where time must be limited to a few seconds the first few times.

I want you to grab life, enjoy life, live every day to its fullest! Use reflexology to stimulate the electrical life force within you!! (Compare using reflex therapy on your body to connecting an electrical lamp with an outlet—the light will not work if there is no electricity flowing through it.) The same is true with your body.

Reflexology is nature's method of electrifying and reinforcing natural energies throughout your entire body and, when used properly, will help you overcome fatigue. Remember we learned in Chapter 2 that the right hand has positive electrical power and is the best for stimulating energy. Use your right hand to tap the top of your head. See Photo 10. Tap your chest (thymus gland reflex) to generate potential strength and activity. See Photo 1. Also, rub fingernails of both hands together to generate renewed energy. See Photo 8.

When toxic fluid gets trapped within the lymph glands, your body will feel fatigued. A vigorous reflex workout to the lymph glands will encourage the removal of waste from your body. See Photo "G" on page 259. New energy pathways will be opened up, as old cells are removed and flushed out of your system. (Remember to drink eight glasses of water every day to help flush out waste.)

As the energy pathways open up, fatigue will dissipate and you will experience an exhilarating liveliness, renewed ambition, and a cheerful enthusiasm for your life.

Doctor Levin, a nutrition specialist, tells us that women with heavy flow and fatigue, could have an iron deficiency, and should take a supplement of folic acid and vitamin B-12. For those who suffer from menstrual pain and breast tenderness, he suggests chewing several dolomite, calcium, and magnesium tablets. Magnesium helps your body absorb calcium more efficiently. Studies show women who take calcium supplements suffer less pain from cramps than those who don't.

USE REFLEXOLOGY BEFORE AND AFTER SURGERY

Reflex therapy is beneficial in stimulating the circulation for natural healing processes both before and after operations. It helps relax and heal. A hysterectomy (removal of uterus, and sometimes ovaries) can leave the body in distress. If the ovaries are removed, the estrogen supply will be diminished. Thus, the adrenal glands must compensate.

Work the reflex to the adrenal gland, thyroid, and pituitary to stimulate needed hormones. A complete workout to all reflex points is strongly advised before and after an operation to benefit good circulation and stimulate the natural healing processes.

Help for Hot Flashes

When your metabolic rate is too high, you may experience a feeling of warmness, even to the degree of perspiring. And at other times the feeling may be one of a strong emotional disturbance and muscle weakness. When this happens, you will want to work the reflex to the thyroid gland, which will help reduce these "hot flashes" by balancing the energy-regulating hormones. These hormones are produced by the thyroid, and when balanced, will regulate your metabolic rate. For best results work *all* the endocrine glands. See Chapter 8.

With the use of reflexology, a healthy diet and daily exercise, you will develop a healthy body that functions efficiently and harmoniously. You will have peace of mind and accept the change of menopause as a new beginning to life—one with vitality, excitement, and joy!

Slow Down Your Breathing

Use this special deep breathing exercise to cool off a hot flash and calm your nerves in any situation. Whether you are at the office or beach or in your car, you will be able to lower the arousal of your central nervous system with deep breathing.

Cut your breathing rate in half by taking slow deep breaths. Count your breaths per minute; if you normally take 12 to 16 breaths each minute, slow down and take 6 to 8 deep breaths per minute. As soon as you feel the flash coming, prepare for it: breathe very slowly and deeply, from your abdomen, and remain relaxed. This slow deep breathing exercise along with a gentle reflexology workout, on your hands or feet, is great if you have a difficult time sleeping; the combination works like a wonderful drug-free sedative.

CHAPTER 19

How to Take Care of and Develop Beautiful Breasts

The breasts are important to a woman's self-confidence. She has been conscious of her breasts from the time she was a child. The breasts represent her femininity, and she watches the development of these organs with pride just as a boy watches the development of his reproductive organs.

Not every woman ends up with the beautiful, full, rounded breasts that she would like to have. By using the magic massage of reflexology, you can have the lovely, full rounded breasts of your youth.

MASSAGING THE BREASTS

Place both your hands on the bare breasts, left hand on left breast, right hand on right breast. Using your hands as cups, fingers pointing toward the breastbone, thumbs pointing up with nipples protruding between the thumb and index fingers, gently massage with a rotary motion as you lift the breasts while sliding the fingers up toward the throat. See Diagram "17A," side 1.

Start with the fingers far enough back so that you can feel the pull on the muscles under the arms. Use a forward lifting massage with each rotation. Do not do this very often, at first, or you will have some pretty sore breasts.

Dr. Popov taught us to use this method of developing the breasts in his rejuvenation center, having us pour sea salts over the breasts as we massaged them.

One young woman there previously had silicone injected into her breasts to make them larger, but she complained that they felt uncomfortable and bothered her a lot. Dr. Popov assured her she would not need the added silicone if she faithfully followed the reflex massage of the breasts as directed.

MASSAGING REFLEXES

When you are massaging reflexes in your neck for a beautiful skin, you are also stimulating hormones to help in the development of the breasts. See Photo 30.

Since the breasts are related to the sex glands, you will be stimulating the breasts even more as you massage the reflexes to the gonads and the endocrine glands as explained in other chapters. See also Diagrams 17A, 17C, and 17D.

Kneading and massaging the breasts with the fingers and palms will enlarge them and help them keep their shape.

REVERSING MASSAGE

Reverse the massage by placing the fingers of the left hand on the breastbone and sliding them under the right breast, working the fingers clear around the breast with an uplifting motion. See Photo 53 on page 187. Do this several times, and use the same massage on the left breast. I learned this technique in the Philippines from a vein doctor.

Place the fingers of the right hand on the breastbone between the breasts as before, but here, follow a vein *under* the breast, pressing on the solid bone. Work the fingers around the breast clear around the outer edge and on up into the fore part of the arm. The next time around, follow this procedure but massage on up toward the outer muscle of the arm. See Diagram "17A," side 2. At first, you may find some very tender spots as you do these breast massages. The doctor claims you are cleaning out old, stagnated blood, and it is true. Very soon you will not find any tender places in or around the breasts. If you should feel any unduly tender spots in the breasts that do not go away, be sure to check with a doctor.

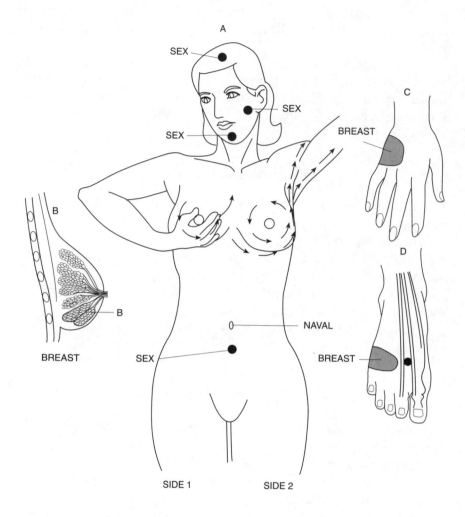

Diagram 17: A shows stimulation areas of the breast, side 1 and side 2. B shows a cross-section of gland and duct. Notice how the lactiferous (milk-producing) glands and ducts flow toward the nipple. C and D show breast reflex pressure points.

Something to remember is that tests in a university study of forty-seven women revealed that 65 percent of the women were able to dissolve their benign breast lumps and avoid biopsy. All they did was alter their diet. According to Dr. John Minton, all that is neces-

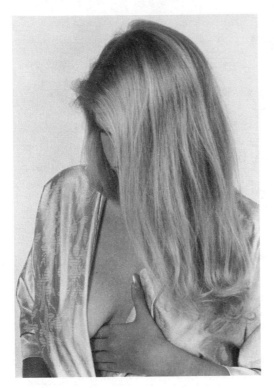

Photo 53: One position for massaging the breast to help develop more beautiful busts.

sary is to give up coffee, tea, chocolate, and cola, which contain stimulants known as methylxanthines. He says that these stimulants provoke the growth of cystic lumps.

Now, one more breast massage:

Place the fingers of the left hand on the nipple of the left breast and slowly massage toward the outer part of the body in a circle. Keep enlarging the circle until you are covering the entire breast. This may be done with the flat of the hand also. Do the other breast the same way.

CHAPTER 20

How to Use Reflexology for Beautiful and Healthy Hair

The health of your hair reflects the health of your body. It is the frame for your face and influences the picture others see, be it beautiful or ordinary. When I used to paint, I would take the finished painting to a frame shop and fit the frame to the picture. It is amazing what a frame will do to bring out the beauty of a painting and how the wrong frame can completely ruin the beauty of the same painting.

ENERGIZING HAIR ROOTS WITH REFLEX STIMULATION

The first thing to do to energize the hair roots is to grab handfuls of hair and pull. Ouch! See Photo 9. Do this over the whole head. As you pull and yank it gently, you will feel as if your head is coming alive. This feeling will last several minutes. Look at Diagrams 12, 13, and 14 to become aware of how many gland and organ reflexes are being stimulated as you do this exercise. This is also said to help a hangover, indigestion, and other complaints.

To further stimulate these reflexes in the head, lightly close your hands into loose fists. With a loose wrist action, lightly pound the whole head. See Photo 10. This will not only stimulate the hair but also the brain, bladder, liver, and many other organs in the body.

Look at Photo 11 where a wire brush is being used to tap the reflexes in the head to add even greater electrical stimulation to the hair and many other parts of the body.

HOW TO ACTIVATE REFLEXES TO THE HAIR

Now, we will turn to the miraculous method of buffing the nails to stimulate hair growth. See Photo 8. Place the fingernails of one hand against the fingernails of the other hand and buff them together. Buff, faster and faster, until you are making them sing. After doing this a few moments, stop and hold the hands relaxed. Feel the buildup of electrical energy in the hands. When you relax, you feel this powerful force stimulating your whole body.

> Mr. D. came to see me after using the nail buffing for a few weeks to regrow hair. Mr. D. told me that he had a very hard time getting up in the mornings. It seemed that his energy had all drained out during the night; he had been this way for many years. Since he was quite bald, he decided to try my suggested method of buffing his nails. He decided that the best time to do this was in the morning before he got out of bed. He would buff his nails for five minutes every morning and then hop out of bed full of pep and energy. One day, it dawned on him that buffing his nails was stimulating not only his hair but his whole body. He says that he has never again had trouble getting up and happily showed me a new growth of hair on his head. He was very proud. He told me about his mother-in-law who was quite elderly. She had very white hair and had tried the same treatment. He said that she had also regained a lot of her old energy but that her pretty white hair was all turning dark on the back of her head.

For beautiful hair, you must keep it clean by shampooing often. Aloe vera and jojoba are very good to help keep the hair beautiful and healthy. Vinegar is still a good rinse. Always wash your comb and brush when you wash your hair, and make sure you use a large comb with wide space between the teeth so that it will not stretch and break the hair. I also use a wire brush, which not only stimulates the hair but tends to go through the hair without disturbing the hairstyle.

Many wonderful letters from readers all over the country have arrived telling me of their success contributed to buffing the fingernails. Here is one of those letters:

Dear Mrs. Carter,

About a year ago, an elderly friend of the family revealed that for years he had been buffing his nails and contributed his abundance of hair to this procedure. His brothers are quite bald.

A friend and I became interested and began looking for more on the subject that led to your excellent books and the section on nail buffing.

In light of the foregoing we thought there may be a place in our society for a mechanical device that would simulate the nail buffing while in the comfort of your armchair watching TV, for example. After many, many hours of trial and error, successes and failures, and so on, we finally accomplished what we set out to do. The next step was a testing program.

A group of thirty participants experiencing hair loss and/or balding, aged twenty to fifty-eight agreed to a daily simulated nail buffing "treatment," which was administered by a lady at a selected location. After three months we were astounded by the reports.

Each and every one noted hair loss stoppage.
Several noted the beginning of hair growth.
Several noted darkening of the gray areas.

We have applied for a patent on our machine and are about to expand on our testing program. We thought you would be interested in this information.

Thank you and keep up the good work.

Sincerely,

—W.R.

STIMULATING HAIR FOLLICLES

Let us look a little further into stimulating the hair follicle. This is for those who have lost their hair and for those who find their hair thinning in certain spots.

Place your first two fingers in front of the upper half of the ears on the bony structure of the head. We know that the hair needs stimulation to be healthy, but mainly it needs blood. You are going to push the blood up into the roots of the hair with your fingertips. Press hard enough to feel the blood being forced up into the scalp. Do this several times, working toward the front and then toward the middle of the head and then around to the back. Start this slowly and not too hard at first or you might start a headache.

ENRICH THE BLOOD FOR VIBRANT HAIR

Work the reflex on the back of your neck to the medulla oblongata (see Diagram 13), which maintains vital body functions such as breathing and circulation. You may wonder what breathing has to do with healthy hair. Breathing provides the oxygen to energize our bodies. When we breathe deeply we enrich the blood with oxygen and energy that is vital to our health and essential to vibrant hair. So remember to breathe deeply and stimulate the medulla oblongata reflex.

Good circulation and healthy blood are essential to our hair, as is water. The blood needs adequate water to flush the system and maintain moist skin and healthy hair.

There are two foods that are excellent for healthy hair growth. One is blackstrap molasses, as it has a high content of iron for rich blood. (Add two or three tablespoons to a small glass of milk, or use it when you bake.) The other is alfalfa, which supplies the blood with chemicals to produce keratin, a substance necessary for forming the principal matter of hair and fingernails. You may need to take this in a tablet form. See page 282 for more about alfalfa.

One reason for hair loss is sluggish hormones and a low level of activity of the pituitary gland or the thyroid gland. You will want to stimulate the reflex to these glands. See Diagrams 2 and 12. The pituitary is known to discharge at least nine hormones, each having a different function. Some examples are controlling kidney function: regulating water balance, skin color, bone, hair and body growth. Make sure to stimulate this internal healer for a healthy hormone balance.

The thyroid controls the body's development and stimulates the activity of your body cells and tissues. And the heart keeps your circulatory system in tip-top condition. So do not neglect the stimulation of this reflex so that you will enjoy better health and great looking hair.

Now you know all there is to know about having a beautiful head of hair. With a diet rich in vitamins and minerals (especially zinc), and lots of vegetables and fruit, you can have the healthiest, most beautiful hair in town.

CHAPTER 21

Treating Coughs and Colds with Reflexology

Colds and flu usually start with a sore throat, so let's cure the sore throat before it turns into something worse.

If I feel the slightest warning of sore throat, the first thing that I do is the lion posture from yoga. This simple posture stops a sore throat before it gets started. See Photo 54. Get down on your knees, sit back on your heels, place the hands on the knees, and spread the fingers as far apart as you can. Inhale a deep breath, and as you exhale the breath, stick out your tongue, straining to reach the chin with the tip of the tongue until you almost gag. Stiffen your fingers and bug your eyes out as you become very tense. Hold this position of tension for a few seconds, then relax. Repeat this posture four or five times, and you will be amazed to feel almost immediate relief from the sore throat. The lion posture rushes an extra supply of blood to the affected area. It tones and strengthens the muscles and ligaments in the throat.

A Yoga Posture Helps a Child

It is truly amazing how quickly this method stops a sore throat for all ages. I had my three-year-old granddaughter do this posture one day when she complained of her throat hurting. We made a game out of the posture and all got on the floor and did it with her. When she got up, she said, "I don't have an ow-ey in my neck anymore, Mommy."

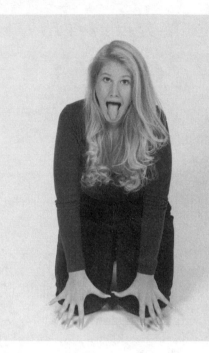

Photo 54: Kneeling position to cure a sore throat.

That was the end of the sore throat. My daughter was amazed even though she had been taught to use this posture since she was a young child. She said, "We get so involved with doctors and advertised drugs, we forget the true and simple healing methods of nature."

Healing in Strange Places

I have taught this posture to many of my friends, some in very odd places—like in the rest room of a large resort. A young woman with a bad sore throat was going to cut her vacation short and go home. She told me, "We planned this vacation for months, went to a lot of work finding the right person to stay with the children, got reservations almost a year ahead, and now, this! We really needed to get away by ourselves for a while. We have a whole two weeks and have only been here two days." I asked her if she would try an odd exercise to help cure the sore throat in a hurry.

I had her put her sweater on the floor to kneel on and showed her how to do the lion posture. She did it several times, and when she got up, she looked at me in amazement. She felt her throat, swallowed a few times, and said it felt completely well. I showed her the reflexes on the feet and the hands, told her to massage any spots that showed tenderness, and advised her to do the lion posture whenever she felt she needed it. I also told her to get some apple cider vinegar if she could. If this was not possible, any kind of vinegar would do. She should dilute it with water and gargle often, swallowing a little each time she gargled.

I don't know when I have ever seen anyone so elated. She hugged me and cried with joy. She said that she would call home and tell her baby-sitter what to do with the children if they developed sore throats. We saw her and her husband several times after that, and they were acting like happy newlyweds.

USING HAND REFLEXES

The reflex for the throat is located on the lower part of the thumb where it fastens onto the hand and all of that area including the web between the fingers. See Photo 35. This also holds true with the reflexes to the throat on the feet. Search for any tender spots anywhere on the big toe where it joins the foot. I have stopped many a sore throat by massaging this particular area. I find this so, especially, on very small children who cannot do the postures and people who are not able to kneel on the floor for the lion posture See Photo 54.

There is healing benefit in apple cider vinegar, especially in destroying germs. In Dr. D. C. Jarvis's book, *Folk Medicine*, he tells of the uses for and cures brought about by applying cider vinegar. One of them is its ability to cure strep throat.

An Unusual Remedy

I brought my eight-year-old granddaughter home to our ranch one summer. Her mother said the girl had been to a doctor for strep throat, but that she had been cured by medication. We were home about two days when I noticed that she was having a hard time swallowing. I looked in her throat and found it covered with white nodules. I knew the strep was back again. I immediately started giving her a mixture of two teaspoons of apple cider vinegar in a glass of water. I had her gargle this every half-hour and swallow a little each time. In a very short time, the throat was clear of all inflammation and the strep germs never returned.

EXPLORING THE TONGUE

Using the tongue probe is also very helpful in curing a sore throat. Just press the back of the tongue with the reflex tongue massager, feeling for tender buttons on the tongue. Some of these can be very sore, but remember what we say in reflexology: "If it hurts, rub it out." Since this is a sensitive reflex area for many malfunctions of the body, be sure to keep a check on any tender spots that might appear on the tongue. See Photo 22.

HELP FOR OTHER SYMPTOMS

Now that we have learned to eliminate one of the first signs of a cold, let us go to the other symptoms, such as sneezing and coughs.

When one has developed a bad cold, it is wise not to give complete reflexology treatments. A cold usually indicates that impurities have accumulated in the system and that the body is trying to clean house by expelling these harmful toxic substances. When we massage certain reflexes, we are helping the body throw off poisons and taxing certain glands and organs, causing them to do extra work in helping the body clean house. So, the only reflexes we will work on during a cold are the pituitary reflex, which is located in the center of the big toe and the thumb, and the throat reflexes. Also, we can press and massage the reflexes to the lungs to help them utilize an added supply of oxygen.

You will see the special reflex buttons for the lungs as you study Diagrams 7 and 8. Press this whole area if you find tender spots on or near the reflex points. Also, search for tender reflexes in the ears and the body warmer buttons on the head. See Diagrams 14 and 15.

If you want to abort a cold before it gets started, take a coffee enema. I have done this many times, and it really works. Use about three teaspoons of instant coffee to a quart of warm water or make a pot of regular coffee and use it. It is said that it stimulates the liver. Do not use a coffee enema at night; it may keep you awake. Use honey instead.

Vinegar and honey are good remedies to take orally, and don't forget the power of the onion and the magic healing properties of garlic. We all know that we must take a large amount of vitamin C to stop a cold or to help get over one quickly. Take a lot of lemons, but not oranges or grapefruit. Massage the pituitary reflexes to lower a fever.

How a Bad Cough Was Stopped Instantly

While I was in a large hotel in Hawaii, I noticed that one of the maids had a very bad cough. She hardly stopped coughing between breaths. When we went out into the hall, I walked up to her and said, "Here, hold your finger like this." I showed her how to squeeze the joint near the end of her middle finger with the fingers of the opposite hand. She looked very puzzled and doubtful until an older Hawaiian maid came and said, "You do what she says, she knows." So the girl did as I told her and she stopped coughing almost immediately.

When we came back several hours later, she greeted me with the greatest enthusiasm—she couldn't thank me enough. There was no sign of the cough that had been troubling her earlier. We were there for several days, and I never heard her cough again.

I hope that you will pass the sensational principle of simple reflex massage on to anyone who might meet with a hard-to-overcome health problem. And then tell them to pass the information on to others. In this way, you will light one more candle to send out healing beams to a sick and suffering world.

Reflexology for Bronchitis

Dear Mrs. Carter,

I know that everything you say in your books is true. I use so many of your methods to help friends and loved ones and myself. I will tell you of one experience I had.

One morning, I got up with a very bad cough. I was gagging and was very sick, so I went to a doctor. After looking at my throat and X-raying my chest, he said I had bronchitis. I informed my father-in-law of my problem and he used reflexology treatments on me as described in your book. I went back to the doctor in a few days and he said that I was well. Now, when I get sick, I go to my father-in-law and he makes me well. Everyone, young and old, should have your reflexology books in their home library.

Thank you.

—Mrs. M.N.

How Reflexology Cures Headaches

Headaches occur for many reasons, some due to a specific health problem such as flu, digestive problems, depression, eyestrain, sinus trouble, hay fever and other allergies, and stress. When using reflexology, you will work on the reflex point that corresponds to the part of the body causing the pain. Millions of people turn to drugs to get temporary relief. Now, you can turn to nature and reflexology and learn sure, quick ways to stop a headache almost immediately. You can do it yourself any place the headache strikes—at home, in the office, at a party, while camping, and so on. Because reflexology tends to heal the whole body by opening up closed electrical lines, it prevents the headache from recurring.

Look at Diagrams 12, 13, and 14. No wonder the head can ache in so many places. Notice all the reflex buttons on the head and face. When you think that each one of these is connected to an electrical channel that leads to some part of your body, you can readily understand why the head can ache.

USING HAND REFLEXES

Let us start with the reflexes in the hands. These are the simplest, easiest reflexes to reach in any emergency. Since the reflexes in the thumbs represent the head area, first massage the thumb reflexes. With the thumb of the opposite hand, start pressing on the center of the pad of the thumb; then squeeze the sides of the thumb by pressing each side of the nail. With a firm pressure, massage just below the thumbnail on top of the thumb, searching for tender buttons. Cover the complete thumb with searching massage; remember, do not rub the skin, but the reflexes *under* the skin. If you don't find a sore spot on one thumb, change hands and give the other thumb the same massage. When you do find an "ouch" spot, massage it for several minutes or until the head stops aching. This works nine times out of ten. See Photo 55.

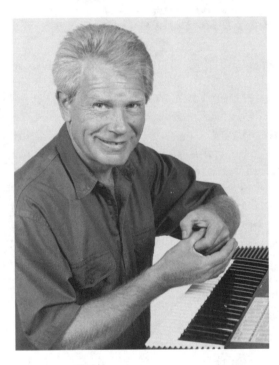

Photo 55: Organist massages reflexes in the thumb to relax nerves and stop a headache.

If the headache persists, place the thumb on the web of the opposite hand between the thumb and forefinger. Pinch and massage this whole area, clear up to where you feel the bones come together, searching for tender buttons. See Diagrams 12A and 12D and Photo 35. This reflex stimulates many parts of the body, so if you find an "ouch" spot here, be sure to rub it out. If you can't find a sore spot here, change hands and do the same to the opposite hand. Since this is one of the crucial reflex buttons for the whole body, it is a good idea to keep this area free from sore spots at all times.

If the headache *still* persists, press and massage the reflexes in the center of both hands, searching for tender buttons. The magic massager will be useful here—it should be used every day to help keep these reflexes stimulated and the electrical life lines open to every part of the body.

USING FOOT REFLEXES

You will find that massaging the reflexes of the feet works miracles, not only for headache but for any other health problem that you might have. Massage all the reflexes in each foot, searching for tender reflex buttons. You may find the reflexes in the feet to be more sensitive than anywhere else on the body. I believe these reflexes in the feet to be most powerful of all in their ability to stimulate the healing life force to every part of your body by opening up closed or clogged electrical lines.

This is why I so highly recommend the reflex foot massager. It is easy to use while you are watching television, talking on the phone, or sitting anywhere. See Photos 42 and 43. It will really stimulate the *healing universal life force* within every part of your body and touch the malfunctioning area that is causing the painful headache. If you haven't already overcome the headache, let us go on to other reflex buttons.

I received a letter from one of my students who was successful in relieving her friend from terrible headache pain. Here is the letter:

Dear Mrs. Carter,

One of my close friends had been to a neurologist and many other doctors, and had many tests to find out how she could cure a very bad headache. Unfortunately, she did not have any success until I was able to persuade her to allow me to work on the inside of her second toe where it joins the foot next to the big toe. After only a few times of working this reflex point, her headache stopped. She is now spreading around the wonderful news of her healing.

God bless and many thanks,

—N.G.

DEALING WITH FREQUENT HEADACHES

Massaging the Head

Look at Diagram 13; see the button called the medulla oblongata at the base of the skull. This button is important in addressing several health complaints that are mainly caused by stress. This is what we call a stress button. Pressing it will bring relief to several health complaints besides a headache. Since its location makes it hard to find and control the pressure needed, it will be more convenient if you use the hand reflex massager. You do not need to press very hard on this particular reflex, just firmly enough to feel the pressure in your head.

Look at Photos 12, 14, 15, 16, and 51 to see how the fingers are being pressed on many areas of the head at once. Use a light but firm pressure as you move the fingers onto different reflexes with a slightly rotating massage. Remember, you are massaging reflexes under the skin, not the skin itself. If you find any reflexes painful to the touch, massage them for a few minutes. Massage the reflexes around the ears, searching for tender reflexes. There is a reflex on the ear that has been known to relieve certain types of headaches. First, you will need to look at Diagram 15, noticing the reflexes to the neck, forehead, and back of head. These basic reflex points are on the cartilage along the back side and bottom of the ear opening. Hold the thumb behind the ear and press your index or middle finger into these points (one finger will reach all points as you move it in a pressing, soothing circular motion). Then press and work the ear lobe, gently if the headache is mild and vigorously if the pain is intense. Keep massaging on down the side of the neck to the shoulders and along the top of the shoulders. See Photo 39. Massage all the muscles in the back of the neck to relieve tension that may be slowing the circulation to the brain, eyes, and other organs within the head. See Photo 13.

Using the Heel of Your Hands for Additional Pressure

If your fingers do not have enough strength to work the reflex points on your head, you may want to use the heel of your hands. Be careful when using this exercise, not to press too hard, as one usually has more strength than they realize when using this type of pressure. You can use the heel of one hand at a time, or you can clasp hands together (see Photo "E") behind your head—using the heels of your hands to work and press the reflex points. You will be able to reach many reflex points with this technique.

Bend Head Forward for Quick Relief

Now I will tell you another quick way to release pressure from the head area. Bend your head forward, working the reflexes on your

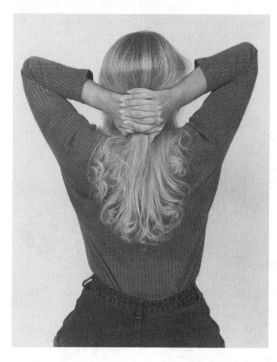

Photo "E": For additional pressure use the heel of hands to stimulate reflexes in back of head.

head. Press lightly over the whole head with your fingers or knuckles, in a slow shampooing motion. Start at the top and work down. If you find tender reflexes, work these points for 15 to 30 seconds, then move on. Go back and forth, covering the entire head—each time you may add additional pressure, but never too hard or you may cause bruising.

Move your hands away from your body and give them a slight shake; this will drain tension away from the head. Repeat twice.

Relieving Headaches Caused by Eyestrain

If eyestrain is causing a headache you will work the reflex buttons for the eyes, which you will find on each foot at the base of the second and third toes or on the hands at the base of the index and middle finger of each hand. See Diagrams 3 and 5.

Another reflex button can be found just above, and on both sides of, the bridge of the nose. Slightly above the eyes, just below the underside of the eyebrow, use middle fingers and simultaneously work buttons.

The most common reflex point on the head is found at the outer side of the eyes, at the temples. Reach up and rub these points simultaneously with your middle fingers. If you have long fingernails, or your fingers are weak, you can use your knuckles. See Photo "F."

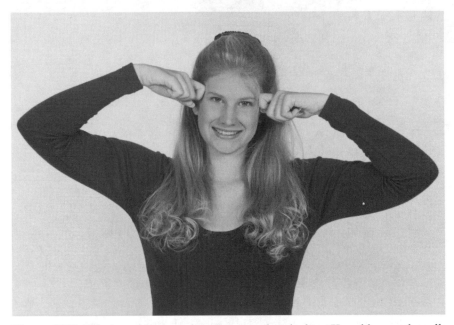

Photo "F": Use knuckles to relieve tension headaches. Knuckles work well for those who have weak fingers or long fingernails.

OTHER METHODS FOR RELIEVING HEADACHES

You may need to change your diet by eating lots of fresh vegetables and fruits, avoiding sugar and chocolate and (for some people) coffee and dairy products. *Don't overeat.* This is the most common sin against health committed by the American people. We eat too much. I can remember people saying that my grandparents didn't eat enough to keep a bird alive. They lived healthy lives to the ages of 99 and 103.

The late Edgar Cayce, told many of his people to sit with the back straight and bring the chin forward to touch the chest, then tilt the head back as far as possible to help open the flow of blood in the pipelines leading to and from the head. I knew a woman who did this one hundred times every day, and she threw away her glasses. Don't do this more than five times at first, or you will develop a headache from tight and sore muscles.

One of the best ways to relieve a headache is to do a lot of walking, especially if you do it in the fresh air. Be sure to wear good shoes. The theory seems to be when we exercise, the lungs process more oxygen, which will increase circulation and ease tension. Aerobics, walking, deep breathing, and reflexology all are good avenues to avoiding tension headaches.

Another person wrote to tell me that the best treatment for them, along with the use of reflexology, is a good fifteen-minute hand or foot soak. She claimed that this always seemed to work for her. This does work for some people, as the hands or feet become hot, the body temperature raises in this area of the body...which ultimately brings the blood flowing down to this part of the body and away from the head to release built-up tension.

I have given you many ways to banish your headaches forever. You will not need to do all these techniques; choose the ones that seem to help you the most, and live the rest of your life free from pain.

HOW TO CURE A MIGRAINE HEADACHE

If you feel that you have what is called a migraine headache, the first thing to do is look for the cause. Many people have suffered for years from terrible headaches, only to discover they were caused by an allergy to a simple household item. Some migraines are caused by the spine or the neck being out of adjustment. Many headaches are caused by additives in food or by air pollution.

I know of many people who have rid themselves of what they called migraine headaches by using the simple method of reflex massage. After you have pressed the reflex buttons on your body, including the reflexes on the hands and feet, search the neck and head for tender buttons that will give you a clue to the cause of your pain. Work on all the reflexes involved. Keep the thymus active by tapping it often, and smile a lot. See Photo 1.

My daughter had terrible headaches for years; the muscles on the back of her neck would tighten up, stopping the circulation of blood to her head. She moved out of the valley into the mountains and her headaches stopped almost completely. When she went to town in the valley, she always came home with a terrible headache. Reflex massage helped, but we couldn't get at the cause until we discovered that the culprit was the smog. It had been causing what we thought were migraine headaches.

You should be able to find the cause and eliminate your headache by testing your reflex buttons and massaging all tenderness out. If the cause is an allergy or additives in your food, then you must eliminate this cause by experimenting.

Especially massage the medulla oblongata at the back of the head. See Diagram 13. Also massage the reflex buttons halfway between the medulla and the ears. See Photo 13. Massage the pain reflexes, the web between the thumb and forefinger (see Photos 35 and "C") and also between the large toe and the second toe. See Diagrams 6A, 6D, and 6E. Massage the reflexes to the stomach on the hands, feet, and body. See Diagrams 3, 5, 7, and 8.

The herb "feverfew" is very effective in stopping migraine headaches for many people. The recommended amount is one tablet, three times a day.

FAINTING OR DIZZY SPELLS

To overcome fainting, you must immediately get your head lower than your heart. When I was pregnant and felt a dizzy spell coming on, I would pretend to fix my shoe and no one noticed that I was stopping a fainting spell. After you get the blood to your head, press hard between your nose and lip. See Photo 46. Press the adrenal reflex button in the center of each hand and also the center of each foot. See Diagram 2. Press your fingernails into the center pad of the thumbs, reflexing the pituitary and pineal glands.

When you have time, check all your reflexes to find the cause of your dizzy spells, and massage them out.

To stop a seizure, grab the thumb and pull it back hard toward the wrist. See Photo 56.

Son Helps Teacher at School

Dear Mrs. Carter,

I want to tell you what my son David, age eleven, did for his teacher while in school.

David's teacher gave the class an assignment and asked them if they would study quietly as he had a terrible headache. David walked quietly up to Mr. J.'s desk and started to gently use pressure on certain reflexes on his head.

We didn't even know he knew how to do this. He had fun watching you when you came to the house and cured his father's headache about a month ago.

Mr. J., his teacher, came to see us that very evening wanting to know what David had done and where he had learned it.

In his words he told us, "I was in so much pain I could hardly stand it. I had taken aspirin with no relief, and suddenly I was aware of a soft touch on my head. I thought for a moment it was an angel touching me. Maybe, I thought, I had died." He laughed. "It seemed my head quit hurting almost instantly. I opened my eyes and there stood David doing all these weird pressures on my head with his fingers. Not only was my headache gone, but I felt physically great. Usually after one of these bouts I feel drained and ill for several hours. David said it was reflexology. I had to come over and learn more about it. I have never had such complete relief in my life."

He thinks David is a natural healer. How can we ever thank you for showing us all these simple natural methods of healing?

—Mrs. J.S.

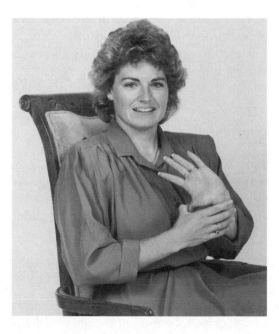

Photo 56: Position for pulling the thumb back to help stop seizure.

CHAPTER 23

How to Use Reflexology to Relieve Back Pain

All practitioners recognize the importance that the spine has in the general health of the whole body. A great part of one's well-being depends on the condition of the spine. The largest percentage of back pain is caused from tension in the muscles that surround the spine. When undue strain is placed on a muscle somewhere in the back area, it tends to tighten and pull on certain vertebrae, causing the spine to be pulled out of alignment. We are all aware that the body can never function in perfect health if the spine is out of alignment.

LOW BACK PAIN IS THE LARGEST SINGLE MEDICAL COMPLAINT IN THE UNITED STATES

Many people in our country have suffered from this painful malady for years. They have gone to doctors and chiropractors without any lasting relief. When they finally searched out a reflexologist who understood the method of massaging the reflexes, in most cases they found permanent relief.

Back Pain Relieved All Over the World

I have received hundreds of letters from all over the world telling of the wonderful relief people have received from painful back problems.

They used the simple but rewarding method of massaging the reflexes to the back that are located on their hands and on their feet. Now we will go a step further and show you how to use this wonderful healing method of massaging reflexes on other parts of the body, which will also bring almost instant relief from back pain.

Back Helped for Good

Dear Mrs. Carter,

I was troubled with painful back muscles for several weeks. Nothing seemed to help for long. One day, I decided I would try a different technique of reflex massage, since it had always helped me for other painful symptoms. I checked my hand with the chart and decided that I had not been massaging in the correct place. The muscles on the right side of my back were affected, so I felt for tender spots on the pad of my right hand below the little finger, and sure enough, I discovered some very tender places. After rubbing them a few minutes, the pain in my back lessened. In three days, all pain and tightness were gone and never returned. It pays to use your own testing along with the help of the charts when a problem doesn't clear up with ordinary directions. I truly believe that there is a reflex someplace that will alleviate pain and eliminate its cause, if we just search for it. I have proved this to be true. Thank you.

—Mrs. J.S.

Relief from Back Pain

Dear Mrs. Carter,

I am a twenty-one-year-old female who is employed in a job that requires me to stand and bend over all day. I have seen several chiropractors, but have not gotten much relief. Last Monday, I could barely walk, move, bend over, or turn my head because my lower back hurt so badly. My friend told me to try reflexology. I was willing to try anything so I went to see Mrs. K., and within fifteen minutes I felt like a new person. That afternoon I was able to shop and do housework, and most important of all I was able to go to work the next day, pain free! I was so happy with the results, I am now a firm believer in reflexology.

—C.N.

Reflexology Brings Instant Relief

Dear Mrs. Carter,

Three weeks ago, one of my students, a young woman in her late twenties, was suffering excruciating pain from an injured back. She dreaded taking the medication the doctor had given her for she suffered ill effects, and would not be able to attend school. I could not touch her in the school environment, so I told her to take off her shoes, and I directed her how to massage the response area to the spine. She had instant relief. She has been attending school every day since then, in perfect health. To me, the best investment I have made is the time I put into studying reflexology. It makes me happy to see the expression of relief and joy on the faces of those who have been restored to health.

—Ms. B.

How to Work the Tender Buttons

Let me explain how to work the reflexes in the hands and the feet to relieve many types of back pain.

You will note in Diagram 5 that the whole spinal column is located in the exact center of the body. Now look to the feet and note that from the big toe on the inside of the foot there is almost a replica of the spine. Follow this area with the fingers or a reflex device as it progresses along the foot to the heel. If you have any weakness in the spine, you will find very tender spots along this area. If the tenderness is near the toe, then the spine is weak between the shoulders. As it progresses toward the heel, you are following the spine down to the tailbone (coccyx). When you work on any of these tender places, you are stimulating a renewed life force into the part of the spine that for some reason is not getting a full supply of energy. When you work these tender buttons on your feet, it is like turning on an electric circuit that has been cut off from its source of power.

In the hands we find the same reflexes to the spine, but our blueprint of the electrical circuit of reflex buttons is moved to the forefinger and the bone that goes from the base of the finger to the wrist. See Photo 57. We also work on the bony structures of the thumb where it joins the wrist. This helps the lower back.

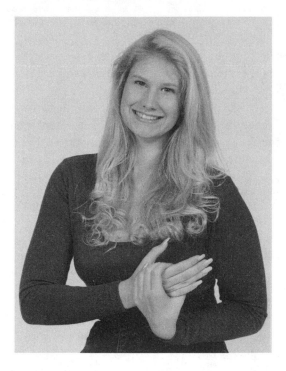

Photo 57: Position for massaging reflexes in the hands to overcome back problems.

Cure in a Few Minutes

Dear Mrs. Carter,

When my brother brought me to you, I was in so much pain from my back I could hardly walk. I had strained my lower back about a week before, and it kept getting worse instead of better. My family finally talked me into going to see you. In just a few minutes my pain was gone after you pressed a few reflexes in my back and then on the backs of my legs. Now any time I have a backache, I have my wife work on these reflexes like you showed us. We can't thank you enough.

—S.M.

WHY OTHER TREATMENTS SOMETIMES FAIL

When muscles are not loose and pliable, they can pull the bones out of place again (after a spinal adjustment) if they remain tight. In most cases, chiropractic adjustment helps, but if the back does not respond to adjustment, turn to reflex massage to relax and loosen up those tight muscles.

All muscles need fresh oxygenated blood and can't respond to nerve impulses without it. Tight muscles are starved for oxygen. So, let us first learn to loosen those muscles. When you massage the muscles to loosen them so that fresh oxygenated blood can flow into them, you are also reopening channels for the flow of life energy to the electrical system. The life force once more flows through all the circuits and brings nature's healing power into play. When you press on certain reflex buttons, you open channels through which the healing forces surge to malfunctioning areas of the body.

MOST CONVENTIONAL TREATMENTS ARE USELESS

When you consider the importance of keeping the muscles pliable and strong, you will understand the harm most conventional methods can cause. A back brace causes muscles to become stiff from lack of normal movement, and traction does not give permanent relief because it doesn't relieve tight muscles. When muscles become too tight over a period of time, they lose circulation, and without adequate blood supply they deteriorate. Drug therapy does nothing for tight hamstring muscles. Then, there is surgery! Even after the expense and suffering, there is still no guarantee that the pain will not return or that you will not become crippled.

Why not try loosening up the tight muscles before you turn to any of these symptomatic treatments? Give reflex massage a chance. Remember, when you are massaging these muscles, to dig in deep with the fingers and rub *across* the muscles, not with them. Loosen them up so that the life force can circulate through them naturally.

Son-in-Law Cured of Low Back Pain

I was visiting my daughter and family not long ago. My son-in-law had been suffering from a back injury for several months. When I visited them, I would give him reflexology treatment and relieve him for the time I was there. They would never follow through with the treatments after I left, so his old problem would return. The last time I visited them, I had him lie on the floor so that I could test the hamstring muscles on the back of the thighs. These were very tight and hard and were painful when massaged. After I loosened up those muscles, his back was free from pain, and he slept like a baby all night.

LOW BACK PAIN IS CAUSED BY TIGHT MUSCLES IN THE HAMSTRINGS

When the hamstring muscles in the backs of the legs become tight, they pull on the pelvis. You can see how this, in turn, pulls on all the muscles and tendons of the lower back. This places pressure on the spine and throws the back out of alignment, causing the discs to slip, rupture, or disintegrate.

Let us now learn how to massage these hamstring muscles to loosen them up and get the oxygenated blood flowing back through them. Sit on the edge of a chair, preferably a straight, hard chair. Relax one leg and place the fingers on the muscles of the thigh on the back of the leg. Press and pull the fingers across the muscles with one hand, then the other. Use the fingers of the other hand to pull across in the opposite direction. Do you feel any hard muscles? Dig in deeper and deeper as you search for a hard, bound muscle. Start at the buttocks and press and pull all the way to where the muscles end at the knee. When you find a hard, tight muscle, massage, press, and pull it. Remember, you are to pull the fingers *across* the muscle, not with it.

When you have finished with this leg, do the same massage on the other one. Remember, if you find any hard, tight muscles in this area, they must be worked out and become soft and pliable when relaxed. Your trouble may be caused by hard tight muscles lying very deep, even those next to the bone, so don't be afraid to massage deep. Work every tight area that you find. It could be quite painful in some cases at first.

If you have someone else to massage the hamstring muscles for you, then lie on a hard table or even the floor. After you get the muscles back to normal, you will find that the reflexes to the back will respond much more quickly, and you will get even better results than you had previously.

Feet Can Cause Back Problems

Some 20 percent of back pain is caused by flat feet. It can be corrected by wearing corrective shoes along with reflex massage. Experiment by wearing different shoes. Many times shoes are the cause of backaches.

Walking Is Beneficial to the Back

Walking is the best exercise for any back problems; it is nature's method of strengthening all the muscles in your body, especially your back muscles. It sends more blood and oxygen to every cell and tissue in your body, including the brain, eyes, and all internal organs. You may walk briskly, but there is no need to run. Jogging has proved to be harmful to 40 percent of those who jog.

A rebounder, which is a small trampoline, will prove to be very beneficial without harming the bone structure of the body and will give you many more benefits than jogging. Vitamin C has been proven to help many a backache.

Straighten Your Back with Foot Exercise

You can correct many ailments with the feet. When I was about seven years old some doctors came through the schools testing our health for various problems. They drew lines down my back and told me it was very crooked. They gave me exercises to do with my feet. In about a month they returned and drew lines on my back again. They were amazed to see how my back had straightened out.

Here are the exercises they gave me: Hold the feet straight out in front of the body, about ten inches apart. Curl the toes back toward the body as far as possible, then bring feet toward each other, so big toes touch. Now force down, holding your toes under as you take twenty steps, walking pigeon-toed. Relax and straighten feet out. Repeat one time then relax feet by shaking each one two or three times.

When you are barefoot, walk briskly around the room, taking four steps walking on toes and four steps walking on heels. Walk a total of twenty steps to strengthen the feet. Sometimes I walk on the outside of my feet, then on the inside. I still do these exercises to keep my back straight and strong.

Stair Climbing

Just a few words about this wonderful exercise. Stair climbing will burn calories and is an excellent workout for the whole body. It works the ankles so the lymphatic system is stimulated to boost the immune system. Your heart and lungs will benefit, comparable to a brisk run, swim, or bike ride. This may reduce stress by channeling it into a positive force. Smiling a very big smile while you exercise will stimulate your thymus.

How Reflexology Helps Back Pain Disappear

Dear Mrs. Carter,

I've learned that reflexology is simple, safe, and effective for anyone, anywhere, anytime. The dynamic healing force of reflexology can make you whole, can bring vigor, vitality, and beauty back into your life, and can help keep you free from illness and pain for the rest of your life if used properly. Reflex massage is therapeutic and can eliminate the cause and symptoms of sickness and pain from the whole body!

One Sunday morning while watching a baseball game on T.V. I felt a sharp pain in my lower back. I took my left foot and massaged the reflex button of the lower lumbar. In a few seconds my back pain suddenly disappeared. I massaged the right foot also. Now I know that reflexology really works.

Aloha and Mahalo!

—Mr. C.S., Hawaii

I Feel Great, Thanks to Reflexology

Dear Mrs. Carter,

I have had back trouble for thirty years. Last year I went to a chiropractor and after thirty treatments was no better, but, in fact, seemingly worse. I was in constant pain. The nights were almost unbearable. I couldn't bend over to brush my teeth without leaning against the cabinet for support. Even coughing was painful. In March I bought *Body Reflexology*, and read what to do for the lower spine. I began reflexology immediately, and that night I slept through without pain. There was instant relief, and it took only about six weeks before all the pain was gone. Although my back is still a little stiff, I feel great thanks to reflexology!

—J.W.

Relief from Back Pain and Sciatic Nerve

Dear Mrs. Carter,

First of all, I want to thank you for introducing me to reflexology. I read all your books. It has helped me cure my back pain and sciatic condition. I feel great and stay that way by using reflexology.

One day while at work one of my co-workers was not feeling very well. He told me his back went out again and he was getting pains down his leg. He told me he was going to see a chiropractor after work. I gently applied pressure to the reflex just below the hip (where the back pocket of his trousers is located). He was immediately relieved.

At lunch time, I gave him another quick reflex treatment. He felt so good that he told me he wasn't going to see the chiropractor after work!

—Mr. D.T.

CHAPTER 24

How to Conquer Arthritis with Reflexology

Arthritis is one of the most disabling and painful illnesses and is suffered by people of all ages, even in our age of miracle advances. Scientists can go to the moon, and they can take pictures of distant planets, but they tell us they still have no cure for the painful, crippling ravages of arthritis.

So let us turn back to the simplicity of nature for help. Let us use the magic of reflexology. I have had such wonderful success in relieving people who are seemingly cursed with this disease that I wish I could tell this wonderful news to every arthritis sufferer in the world. I am making some progress in spreading this news, as I receive many letters almost every day from grateful people from most every country in the world who have used my other reflexology books. They thank me for my guidance in bringing them unbelievable relief.

How Mr. A. Helped Himself and Family

Mrs. Carter:

May God bless you forever for the new hope that your wonderful book has given to me and my family. Arthritis seems to run in our family, and doctors have told us there was nothing they could do except give us drugs, which bring little or no relief. I could stand the suffering for myself, but to watch it attack my little children one by one has been the hardest for me to bear.

One day a friend loaned me your book *Helping Yourself with Foot Reflexology.* I started to massage my feet and almost immediately felt the difference in my body. It was like I had suddenly gotten a recharge for a worn-out battery.

I immediately went to work on my children's feet. Even though it was very painful to them, they seemed to realize that some miracle of nature was at work. I am recovering very rapidly. Every day I am better and have a feeling of magnetic vigor that I haven't felt for years. My children are almost back to normal and can once again play with other children. Thanks to reflexology and the Divine Protector we have found new health.

—Mr. A

CHILDREN CAN GIVE TREATMENTS

Children seem to turn instinctively to reflexology once it has been introduced to them. I know children who love to work on the feet of their parents and each other, finding the tender reflexes and relating which gland in the body corresponds to each reflex. My books on reflexology are used in many youth camps, and reflexology is taught and practiced by many Boy Scout, Campfire Girl, 4-H, and other youth groups.

VITAMIN C, BACTERIA, AND ARTHRITIS

Lack of vitamins also plays a large part in the development of arthritis. Scientists have found that by depriving animals of vitamin C over a period of weeks and then introducing bacteria into them, arthritis was produced. The bacteria were carried by the bloodstream throughout the body and lodged in the small joints first. Then the body tried desperately to stop the infection by depositing calcium all around it. Arthritic stiffness, pain, and swelling resulted. When bacteria were injected into animals that were on balanced diets with plenty of vitamin C, the bacteria did not enter the bloodstream but formed an abscess at the point of infection. The abscess and the bacteria drained off.

NEVER ACCEPT DEFEAT

I do not want you to accept defeat in regard to any *seemingly* hopeless ailment. Not even to so serious a problem as arthritis. There is always hope! At this point, learn what to do to relieve the ravages of painful arthritis, maybe for yourself, or a loved one, or a friend. Let us turn to the magic of pressing special reflex buttons to awaken healing electrical life force to all areas of the degenerated joint tissues which have been caused by nutritional deficiencies and other problems throughout the years.

HOW TO USE DEEP MUSCLE THERAPY FOR ARTHRITIS

In Canada a woman has been curing arthritis patients for years with what she calls muscle therapy. Therese Pfrimmer discovered this technique by curing herself after becoming paralyzed from the waist down. She tells us that there is no such thing as a *dead* muscle or nerve. The muscles become tight from overwork. They become tense, the blood supply shuts off, and the muscles become sealed off from the rest of the circulation.

This theory is not unlike reflex massage except that you dig in deeper, reaching through to the very muscles that lie against the bone in many cases. Sometimes these muscles will feel like hard rocks that cannot be brought back to life. But all they need is to receive the circulation of blood back into them, and they will return to normal, and you will be free from the ravages of painful and crippling disease.

MUSCLES, NOT NERVES, CAUSE CRIPPLING

Muscles should be soft and supple, but in tests of the muscle tone of paralyzed people certain muscles are found to be tough, dry, and hardened; the muscle fibers are stuck together and can't be separated. Therese Pfrimmer says that the crippling problems are in the muscles and not the nerves. Paralysis sets in because the muscles become sealed off from the bloodstream. When fresh oxygenated arterial blood is sealed off, the muscles start to degenerate and become hardened. The muscles are also cut off from the flow of lymph—a fluid that lubricates the muscles and keeps them from sticking to each other. Without lymph there is friction and different muscles that should be free and able to move separately stick together.

Deep muscle therapy can be used for seemingly incurable illnesses. It can be used along with reflex massage to bring faster and even more rewarding results, especially in cases where the muscles have become degenerated. I believe that no muscle or nerve is ever dead; it is just strangled by lack of circulation and *can* be brought back to life and health by releasing the flow of lymph and blood back into it. But exercise and physical therapy alone cannot cure a crippling condition where muscles have become hardened. They must be massaged, and the massage must be done in a certain way.

Suppose some of the muscles have been deprived of a supply of vital electrical energy for a long time. The blood supply has slowly been lessened to certain areas of the body. The muscles have become less and less pliable and more painful. When the muscles cannot move a joint, pain and inflammation occur because the muscles are pulling on the joint tissues. When you release the muscles, the joint will repair itself, and pain and stiffness will disappear. In cases such as this, it is often too late for reflexology alone to benefit, so we will turn to the sensational healing principle of deep muscle massage.

How Deep Muscle Massage Helps Arthritis

Here we will deviate a little from the way I have instructed you to use reflex massage. To help get the circulation back into degenerated muscles, we are going to have to reach in deep and massage them back to life. I believe that no muscle or nerve is *dead* as long as you are *alive*. But, after years of being denied the life-giving flow of blood and lymph, they may have become hard and fibrous. To get these muscles back into their natural state of pliability, we must massage them back to life. In some cases, it may not be easy and it may take time to get complete relief, but it will be worth your effort. In many cases, you will feel results almost immediately.

Now, to start using the muscle massage you will press with the fingers wherever the arthritis is bothering you. Take the fingers and press into or near the affected area of the arms or the legs or other parts of the body. Are the muscles soft and pliable, or are they hard against the bone? To massage these areas correctly, dig the fingers into the flesh and reach the muscle lying against the bone, if that is where it feels tight and hard. Start kneading across the muscles—not with them but across them, as if you were pulling across the strings of a guitar, only with a deep massaging motion. This may be painful, but it is the only way to get the flow of blood back into muscles that have become badly degenerated.

Therese Pfrimmer tells us that we must work on the second and third layers of muscles, not just the muscles lying under the skin which are usually treated by regular massage. Remember, we are not just pressing buttons here as in the technique of reflex massage.

THE IMPORTANCE OF THE ENDOCRINE SYSTEM

We look to the endocrine glands in treating the underlying cause of arthritis. When any one or more of these glands are not functioning to their full capacity, there is trouble elsewhere in the body. Look again at Diagram 2; then turn to Diagram 12 and notice where the endocrine reflexes are on the head. You will find the reflexes to the pituitary and the pineal glands located in the center of the forehead and under the nose. Gonad (sex gland) reflexes are at the top of the head and the center of the chin. The adrenal and pancreas reflexes are also located near the top of the head. Also see the reflex buttons to the triple warmer reflexes shown in Diagram 14.

Using all the fingers as shown in Photos 12, 14, 15, and 16, press these reflexes with a steady pressure, holding to a slow count of seven. Now, with the middle finger of each hand, press and massage each reflex button that feels sensitive to the touch. Try to follow the reflexes illustrated on the diagrams as much as possible.

Now, let us look at Diagrams 7 and 8 showing the location of the endocrine reflexes on the body. Press these with the fingers or a hand reflex massager, or stimulate a lot of these by using the helpful reflex roller.

HOW TO STIMULATE NATURAL CORTISONE

Cortisone is a drug used to stop pain. When we massage the reflexes to certain glands, we stimulate these glands into releasing a form of *natural* cortisone into the bloodstream. We are all aware of the damaging side effects that synthetic cortisone has on the body when it is injected. The natural cortisone produced by our glands alleviates pain quickly without any harmful side effects.

Review Diagram 6. Notice a point between the first and the second lumbar vertebrae near the lower part of the back. Press this point, using a gentle pressure to start, increasing it gradually for about seven seconds. This will cause a gland to secrete a natural human cortisone.

Most of you will not know exactly where the first and second lumbar vertebrae are located, but if you start by placing your fingers on the tailbone and then pressing gently on each vertebra, you will feel a very sensitive spot about three fingers' width up from the end of the spine. Use a press-and-hold on this, about three times, and your pain will vanish as if by magic. You may use this for any ailment in which cortisone is helpful. This is especially good for arthritis in various parts of the body, as well as asthma and bursitis.

Bursitis Alleviated

Dear Mrs. Carter,

Reflexology is the most wonderful and natural way of healing I ever dreamed of. I have been taking these treatments for about five years and have been giving them for over two years to friends and neighbors. What really made a believer out of me was this: I had bursitis in my shoulder and I had two pins in one ankle for over twenty years. The ankle was very sore. I had lots of pain and swelling. After two treatments my shoulder was fine, and after three treatments my ankle was much better. Now I have no trouble with bursitis at all.

—Mrs. N.P.

Another Arthritis Sufferer Helped

Dear Mrs. Carter,

I want to tell you of the wonderful results I have gotten from reflexology.

I had arthritis ever since I was seventeen years old and now I am forty-six years old; this is the first time that I am without pain. Plus, my husband was losing all his hair and after doing the hand reflexology as you directed, his hair stopped falling out and is now growing back. I want to thank you very much, and God bless you.

—I.A.

Reflexology Helps Woman Walk

Dear Mrs. Carter,

Gladys came to my office when she could hardly walk. I had to help her into my office and onto the chair. I then applied reflexology to her feet. She almost jumped off the chair when I very lightly touched the reflexes in her left foot at her throat-neck and thyroid reflex. She also had some lower back pain which was fully relieved by the reflexology treatment. After only thirty minutes, the lady walked out of my office...pain free. I've followed up on her condition several times since then, and she is still pain free.

Before coming to my office, she had seen two doctors and had lost three weeks' work. She had been diagnosed as having rheumatoid arthritis and was given some pills that had not helped her.

She is now back at work well and happy. I had never met Gladys before. I invited her to my fiftieth wedding anniversary ceremony this past April. All her family attended. We had a wonderful celebration.

Yours very respectfully,

—J.A.

SPECIAL REFLEXES FOR HIP AND SCIATICA

To relieve many types of pain in the legs and the hips, press on the reflexes around the hip socket. For arthritis pain, search for a very tender reflex on the outer edge of the buttocks.

Since everyone's body is different, you will have to search for these tender reflexes. You may find several sore buttons in this area. When you press on an "ouch" reflex, hold pressure on it as you have been directed to when massaging other reflex buttons. Using the reflex roller massager will be helpful here in locating the tender reflex buttons.

For sciatica pain, which can be excruciating, look first to the pad in your heel. You will probably have to use the reflex hand probe or another blunt device for this reflex button. If your problem is from sciatica, you will have no trouble locating the sore spot in the heel pad. It will be very painful, but by holding pressure on it or massaging it, you will be relieved of all sciatica pain.

Now turn to another reflex to relieve sciatica near the hip joint. Move the leg and find where the hip socket moves; press around in this area until you find a very tender button. Press and hold this with the thumb or finger. It will feel as if you are holding a red-hot poker into your hip, but it will relieve the pain of your sciatica.

Massage Brings Comfort

Dear Mrs. Carter,

Since he got bacterial meningitis my husband has gone steadily downhill. We were at a dead end with doctors. Two weeks ago I started to use reflexology. Four days ago he started to be able to reach the back of his neck with both arms. He had not been able to do this for over two years. His color is better and his depression has much improved. His whole system seems now to be on the mend. Until reflexology I really feared for his sanity. Thanks to God, good food, vitamins, common sense, and reflexology, we are now in better health than we have been in years. God bless you.

—C.U.D.

Dear Mrs. Carter,

I have had low blood sugar for several years. I have never really known that glowing feeling of good health. Then I found your book on reflexology, and by using the method described, I do feel much better. Lately I have had some bouts with arthritis, and then after studying your book I discovered that the two ailments are interrelated. The massage and the clamps have brought immeasurable comfort and ease. I am still looking for a panacea for an abundance of pep and I hope to attain it with the help of the magic massagers.

—G.A.R.

REFLEXOLOGY FOR THE KNEES

I have had many people come to me with painful knees. It seems that for no known reason the knees become painful, and nothing seems to bring relief. But they have never tried the miracle power of using reflexology to cure their knee problems.

A Dancer's Problem Solved

I was at a dance not long ago where a friend kept wanting me to dance with her husband. She finally told me that she was having trouble with her knees and that they were becoming worse all the time. She was afraid that they might have to give up square dancing, which was their main source of exercise. I laid my hand on her knee and pressed with the thumb and middle finger about two inches above the kneecap for a few seconds. She was amazed to find the pain gone, and she danced the rest of the evening. I talked to her several days later. When asked about her knees, she admitted she had forgotten she ever had a problem with her knees.

Before I learned of reflexology, I used to use hot vinegar packs to stop knee pain. These can also be used in conjunction with the reflexology treatment, if needed. So far, I have not known anyone to need further treatment for painful knees after a correct reflexology treatment—pressing the reflex buttons above and below the knees. See Diagram 6C and Photos 58 and 59.

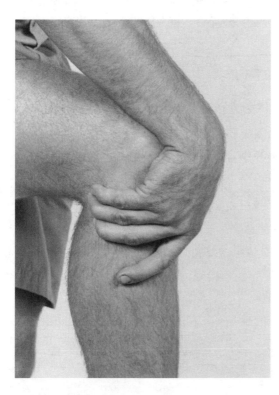

Photo 58: Position for pressing reflexes below the knee to alleviate pain in the knee.

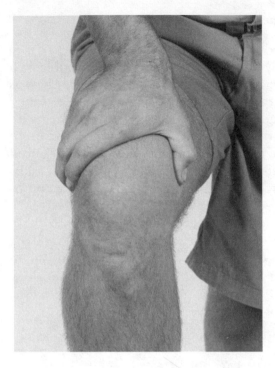

Photo 59: Position for pressing fingers into reflexes to stop pain in knee.

The Function of Your Knees

Did you ever take time to think how much work the knees do? They are truly an intricate marvel of God's design, as is our whole body. No wonder that sometimes these overused parts seem to wear down, which is especially true with athletes. They should all learn to send a renewed electrical supply to weakening areas. By knowing what buttons to press to open up a larger supply of energy and renew the life force into the malfunctioning knee, a person can enable it to return to normal.

Quick Relief for a Knee Problem

My son-in-law told me how much he had been suffering from pain in his knees when I was visiting last year. Since he works mainly at a desk, his problem was not caused by too much exercise (maybe by not enough exercise). I walked over to where he was sitting rubbing his knees, laid my hand on one knee, and pressed with my thumb and finger just above the kneecap for about seven seconds. Then I pressed on the reflexes just below the kneecap for the same amount of time.

I used this method on both knees, and he couldn't believe that they had stopped hurting. I showed him how to do this on himself if the trouble came back. That was well over a year ago. He has not had to use the reflex massage on himself because his knees have never hurt him since the one treatment.

How to Massage Knee Reflexes

To give yourself a treatment for painful knees, take the thumb and middle finger of the right hand, and, just above the knee bone on each side of the right knee where the bone ends, feel a soft spot. It will probably be quite tender when pressed. Now press and hold this with as much pressure as you can stand for about seven seconds.

Now go to the reflex buttons below the knee. You will do the same pressing and feeling as you did above the knee. Find the soft spot or indentation just below the knee bone with the thumb and middle finger. This will probably be quite tender. Press and hold for about seven seconds. Follow the same procedure on the left knee. This is usually all you need to do to end pain in the knees.

Arthritis and Headaches Stopped

Dear Mrs. Carter,

I have been using reflexology on myself for over a year now with wonderful results. I have been diagnosed as having arthritis of the spine and after reflexology, I have been able to quit taking all medication and have not needed it for over a year now. Plus, it has stopped headaches and many other general aches and pains. Thank you so much.

Sincerely,

—D.B.

For Added Pressure

If you have very little strength in your fingers, you can double your pressure by placing your middle finger on top of your index finger. You will be surprised at the added strength this gives.

CHAPTER 25

How Reflexology Helps Carpal Tunnel Pain

Carpal tunnel syndrome, or CTS, can be a very painful disorder, which is caused by stressful, repetitive hand motions. CTS often occurs when tendons in the wrist become swollen and compress the median nerve that runs through the "carpal tunnel" in the wrist and fingertips. As the tendons become swollen from overuse, the nerves that control the thumb and fingers get squeezed, and become weak. As the nerves become weaker, they stop working. This can cause painful burning, tingling, and numbness.

The first thing you will want to do is release the tension in your hand and wrist by relaxing your hands. Find the solar plexus point in the centerpoint of each hand. See Diagram 3. Using the opposite hand, wrap fingers around back and place thumb on centerpoint. (Here is the solar plexus button, which is a potent reflex that calms a network of nerves.) When a pinching, pressing motion is applied to this point, it will help relax the whole body and will help ease the suffering of CTS.

As you press this point, slowly breathe air into your lungs. Hold to the count of seven. Now slowly ease up on the pressure and at the same time slowly release the air from your lungs. Repeat three times on each hand.

If your hand is swollen or sore, it may be to your advantage to work the "referral area," which is the solar plexus reflex on your foot. See Photo "B" and Diagram 5.

HOW TO USE REFLEX POINTS TO EASE PAIN

Work all around the wrist between hand and forearm to open up channels within the tendons for better circulation. You will find there is a pressure point at the flexion crease of the wrist, on the front and back side of the arm. This point is in the middle of the crease and can be pressed from both front and back simultaneously.

This will open up circulation through the tendons to help release swelling and, at the same time, will encourage lubricating fluids to travel through the carpal (*carpal* means "wrist") ligaments to ease the pain. Now move up the arm to another reflex point, which can be found three inches up from the wrist. You can find this reflex by placing three fingers next to the wrist where it bends, on the elbow side of your fingers is the reflex point. Here you can press on the front and back of arm, simultaneously. Hold for seven seconds, then release seven seconds. Repeat ten times, several times a day. Work both right and left wrists for complete circulation. See Photo 38.

I have found through treating CTS that the further one works up the arm and around the back, including all around the shoulders and neck, the better our success of total healing. You can find reflex points that release tension in the carpal (wrist) way up on top of the shoulder. Raise your arm up; now feel toward the outside edge of your shoulder. Here you will find a point that feels hollow, formed at the extreme outer edge of the shoulder. Press into this hollow point for seven seconds, working with a circular pressing motion, and also work up to, and include the neck.

When tension is in the shoulder, it is beneficial to work all the way down and over to the third and fourth points along the spine (see Diagram 18B) and over to just above the shoulder blade. Press and work these reflex points gently at first, then add pressure.

You can also find relief from pain by pressing the reflex button found between the web of your thumb and index finger. Use a pinching or press-and-squeeze motion to work this reflex for a minute or two. Repeat as necessary. See Photo "C".

This button is also excellent for helping those who suffer from rheumatoid arthritis.

How Mrs. A. Was Saved from CTS Surgery

Mrs. A. had very strong pains in her wrists and hands, and at night she would wake up with numbness in them and a tingle, like they had fallen asleep, but she couldn't wake them up. This had to be taken care of, so she called her doctor, and he told her that she had CTS and needed to have both hands operated on.

Mrs. A. could no longer work with such pain, so she made plans for the operation. The day before the surgery was scheduled to take place, Mrs. A.'s daughter came for a visit and asked if she could try to relieve the pain for the night by using reflexology. Mrs. A. knew it would not hurt, and in fact, she had read that reflexology was beneficial before surgery to get the circulation going to speed up healing.

Mrs. A.'s daughter worked her mother's hands, going up her arm, her shoulders, and around her back. On Mrs. A.'s back was a lump, sort of like a swollen muscle, just above the shoulder blade. She rubbed the lump and all around each shoulder blade, gave her mother a kiss and wished her a good night's sleep.

In the morning Mrs. A. awoke with no numbness or tingling, and the stiffness and pain had subsided. When her daughter woke up, Mrs. A. told her that the pain was gone. They talked it over and decided to cancel the surgery. Now Mrs. A. knows what to do when the pain returns. She uses reflexology and some preventive exercises. She never did have the surgery and is very grateful for the wonders of reflexology.

Another friend of mine who makes dolls started getting the symptoms of CTS. Her work is very tedious, as she is a perfectionist and spends hours producing her creations. I gave her a ball so that she could strengthen and exercise her fingers. I worked the reflexes on her hand, arm, and shoulder, up to and around her shoulder blade, where we found it to be very sore. (This is a key reflex point to controlling the pain of CTS. Work the whole area around the shoulder blade, searching for a tender spot; then concentrate on that reflex for several minutes to revitalize the flow of healing energy to your hands.)

Using reflexology and a wrist splint at night, my friend now continues to make beautiful dolls. She approaches her craft with eagerness and is delighted to be able to work with greater ease.

A surgeon in Sitka, Alaska, Dr. John Totten, tells us that fishermen frequently come to him in the middle of salmon season complaining of chronic pain and numbness in their hands. He tells them cortisone injections into the wrist will give them immediate relief, but when used too often, he warns, the shots will cause additional problems.

With the use of reflexology we can release natural cortisone into the bloodstream to alleviate pain, and we will avoid suffering any dangerous effects from drugs. See Diagram 6.

TAKE A BREAK TO AVOID
CARPAL TUNNEL SYNDROME

Work managers need to be aware that employees work more efficiently when they are relaxed, comfortable, and free of pain. The very best treatment for CTS is preventive care. If you are at work, try to prevent wrist problems by moving or stretching every hour, even if it is just for a minute or two. If you are sitting, you will want to keep your feet on the floor, (do not cross your legs) and keep your back straight (do not bend over) so that you will not hinder the proper body circulation. If you're standing, take a break and sit down. Rest the carpal ligaments by working the reflex points to release tension, and try one or two of the following exercises.

Elevation of Hand

If you feel a burning pain from your wrists into the fingers, or if you are awakened at night because your hands have fallen asleep, elevate your hand to eliminate pain. (We know there is swelling of the tissues inside the tunnel walls that are pressing against the median nerve in the wrist.) If you notice swelling in the soft tissue, this exercise is especially helpful.

Strengthen and Exercise Fingers

With fingers all opened and fanned out, bend one finger down at a time, to make a fist, starting with your pinky. Now reopen hand and repeat seven times. Shake each hand vigorously to get the circulation moving. This exercise can also be done around a small ball.

Release Swelling and Irritation in Tendons

Placing right hand under fingers of left hand, gently bend all fingers of left hand backward toward top of left wrist, release, and repeat seven times; then alternate hands. Most often hands and fingers are in a forward position. This exercise will give them relief, and open channels for better circulation.

Stretch the Forearm

Sit in a chair with your back straight, place hands next to your legs, palms of hands flat on seat of chair, with thumb to the outside and fingers pointed backward (toward the back of chair). Now slowly lean your upper torso back to stretch your forearms. (This will hurt, so do not overpull the tendons.) Keep palms flat on chair. Hold for seven seconds, release...repeat twice.

Release Tension

Release tension in hand and wrist by standing and placing your open hands flat on a table, with palms down and fingers pointed away from you, keeping arms straight. Lean your upper body forward, gently pressing your hands against the tabletop, stretching fingers and wrist. Hold for seven seconds. Repeat.

Use a Splint

Place your forearm in a splint to extend your wrist for increased circulation. If the hand is turned upward and the wrist is not bent, blood can flow more freely.

VITAMIN B-6 RELIEVES CTS

Studies show that taking 50 to 200 milligrams of vitamin B-6 daily for three or four months will relieve carpal tunnel symptoms. Dr. John Ellis of Mount Pleasant, Texas, tells us this vitamin will reduce swelling of the tendons that are compressing the median nerve and is known to stimulate the body's natural cortisone. He claims that in twenty-eight years of practice, he's had only five patients who needed surgery after taking vitamin B-6 daily.

You can add natural foods to your daily diet that are rich in vitamin B-6 such as brewer's yeast, bran cereal, brown rice, whole wheat foods, royal jelly, alfalfa, wheat germ, sunflower seeds, tuna, beans, oats, chicken, bananas, and blackstrap molasses, to name a few.

Reflexology is NOT meant to take the place of your regular physician. Many doctors are now including the natural methods of healing in their practice. If your situation is precarious and, at times, seems hopeless, let your instinct of self-preservation tell you not to give up. Here are a couple of cases where reflexology helped when all else failed.

Mr. R. had been to several specialists for help with his inflammation and chronic wrist pain. He was told surgery would help. However, he did not consent to this because he was scheduled for a golf tournament the following Spring. He knew he needed help, as his job put constant demands on the musculoskeletal anatomy which in turn caused weakness in his grip and numbness in his fingers.

His wife said, "Lets try Nature's way to relax tension, so that natural healing can take place." She used finger pressure on his hands, wrist, forearm, shoulders, neck and back. She also included foot reflexology sessions, elevated the extremity, used ice, gave him B-complex vitamins and vitamin C, and kept his diet healthy. . . . That very spring he competed in the golf tournament and now experiences the joys of natural health.

Reflexology Makes Life Worth Living

Dear Mrs. Carter,

I had a severe problem with my sciatic nerve in my right leg. I made fourteen visits to the chiropractor and found no relief. My family doctor put me in the hospital for bed rest and traction. Still no help. Next I was sent to a nerve surgeon and underwent eleven types of tests. Nothing wrong. Next the bone doctors made numerous X-rays and bone scans. After three months in two hospitals, I was released with my problem unsolved, hurting more than ever.

A friend visited me in the hospital and told me about someone who practiced reflexology. I made an appointment and to...my surprise, the third treatment brought me relief!

This was a miracle in my life! This created a great interest on my part and since then I have continued treatments on a regular basis. I know that it is "God sent" and now I want the whole world to know about this simple way to stop those pains and help you to enjoy good health and make life worth living!

—A.M.L.

CHAPTER 26

How to Cure Hemorrhoids with Reflexology

The pain of hemorrhoids can be almost unbearable at times and also very embarrassing. Yet, with the simple technique of massaging certain reflex buttons, I have relieved hundreds of people permanently of this painful affliction. You can heal yourself by just pressing a few "ouch" buttons and feel the pain vanish like magic under your fingertips almost immediately. If you keep up the massage for several days, the hemorrhoids will disappear completely.

Hemorrhoids are varicose blood veins in or around the rectum. To find the reflexes to these troublesome and painful areas, first look to the feet.

USING FOOT REFLEXES

With the finger and the thumb, press on the bony part of the heel, just above the pad. You will find a ridge along this area. Press all the way around this ridge, searching for tender points. See Diagrams 4 and 5. You may have to use a reflex device to help you press hard enough to really massage the reflexes. The hand reflex massager seems to work well here. You will probably not find this whole area tender, just certain points. The swollen veins in the rectum causing the painful hemorrhoids are usually in one or two places. You have to

234

search out the "ouch" buttons and press and massage for several minutes. Sometimes these can be very painful, so start out with as much pressure as you can stand. Now, work your fingers slowly up under the inner anklebonc, pressing firmly, searching for "ouch" spots. Press and massage all along the back part of the leg with the fingers and the thumb on each side of the Achilles tendon. You may find several tender reflex buttons in this area. Don't be afraid to massage them out no matter how painful it may be. Do this complete massage on both feet and legs. Also, check for a tender reflex behind the nails of the big toes.

USING HAND REFLEXES

We will turn to the reflexes in the hand to alleviate the pain of hemorrhoids. Press on the bony part of your wrist with the thumb of the opposite hand. Start on the palm side and press all the areas on or below these bony areas; turn the hand over and press with the thumb or the fingers on the top of the wrist, still searching for the tender reflexes to the hemorrhoids. See Diagram 6A and Photo 38. Do this on both wrists. I have seen this technique completely heal some very bad hemorrhoid cases of long standing. There is also a reflex button on the end of the tailbone. Test this for tenderness also and massage it.

REFLEXES OF THE HEEL PAD

Another very important area of reflexes to the rectum area is located under the pad of the heels. If you have pain in any part of the rectum or lower colon area, you will find these reflexes so tender that you can hardly bear to massage them. Massage them you must, to relieve pain and get the flow of the electrical life force circulating into the problem area so as to help nature heal the inflamed, aching tissues. Remember, when any stimulation is applied to the surface of the body, a reaction will occur somewhere. This is a hard area to reach with the fingers, especially if the foot is callused, so you will probably have to resort to a device to help you reach these special reflexes.

You may first want to try your fingers as shown in Photo 45. Take the pad of the heel in the hand and try to press the tips of the fingers under the pad. If this does not get results, try the hand reflex massager or the reflex comb. Grasping the comb in both hands, roll it from side to side, giving special attention to the area that is located on the inside of the foot, up toward the ankle. This you may find extremely tender. Another way to massage these hard-to-reach reflexes is to use the rung of a chair or table. I discovered these important reflexes on the edge of my coffee table. Use whatever comes naturally until you get the soreness worked out. When the hurt stops in these reflexes, you will find that the hurt in the lower rectum area has also subsided.

Fantastic Improvement

Dear Mrs. Carter,

I have learned from firsthand experience that reflexology most definitely is fantastic for the treatment of hemorrhoids! As a result of an awkward situation, I fell, causing a vein to slightly protrude externally. After the first treatment the soreness was completely gone and the swelling was much improved. With just a few treatments I am back to normal.

—F.S.

Correct Reflex is Important

Dear Mrs. Carter,

I have learned the most important information concerning the reflexes for hemorrhoids! The reflexes on the inside of the foot had not helped my bleeding rectum, but just one spot on each foot on the top of the heelbone on the outside of the foot brought the bleeding under control in three treatments.

Thank you, Mildred Carter, for sharing your knowledge and experience!

—L.T.

Mrs. J.'s Story

Dear Mrs. Carter,

I have had a history of colon trouble for several years, as I told you earlier on the phone. I was visiting for several weeks and couldn't follow my diet. I began suffering terrible pain in the whole lower part of my body. I didn't want to bother anyone with my troubles, but I wasn't very jolly company. At night, the pain was terrible; I just lay there and suffered. Even aspirin didn't help. That is when I decided to call you, and you told me about the heel technique. Now I want to tell you what a godsend your advice was. That evening while everyone was watching television, I started massaging under the pad of my heel. I don't know when I ever had anything hurt that bad. Believe me, it took willpower to keep it up, but I knew I was really on to something when it hurt that bad! I only had my fingers to massage with, but I sat there all evening massaging under the heel pads. One foot was much sorer than the other, so I concentrated mostly on that foot. By the time we went to bed, a lot of the soreness was worked out, and would you believe that I slept all night without pain! I still do not have trouble in this area, and I cannot find any sore spots in the reflexes under my heel pads. I can't praise you enough for sending me the blessing of reflexology.

—R.J.

How Reflexology Relieves Asthma

Asthma is truly a dreadful disease, causing many frightening experiences for the sufferer. When you cannot breathe, your whole body is in trouble. Breath is life; many asthma sufferers die from lack of air in the lungs as well as side effects from the medication that is given for its relief.

An Asthmatic Recovers

A girl who worked for me suffered from asthma attacks that kept getting worse as time passed. Doctors were giving her medication that was very harmful to her body. Doctor J. told her that eventually the medication would kill her.

After a few costly stays in the hospital, she agreed to try reflexology. I sent her to one of my reflexology students who had become very proficient. After very few treatments, she started to improve. At this date she is almost completely recovered. I also recommended that she take vitamins. They helped the body rebuild itself after the years of abuse it had suffered from the ravages of the asthma and the poisonous medications she had been taking.

USING BODY REFLEXES FOR ASTHMA

Now we turn to the reflexes in the body that can help stop an asthma attack. Four important positions will activate your electric lines, sending a surge of healing energy to the congested area causing the attack.

Look at Photo 60. Notice how the finger is pressed into the lower part of the neck. See in Diagrams 18A and 18C how the collar bones form a "V." Place the middle or index finger into this "V" and pull down while pressing firmly inward. Hold a few seconds, then massage downward. Do not press hard enough to bruise. This method is valuable in bringing quick relief from an attack of asthma.

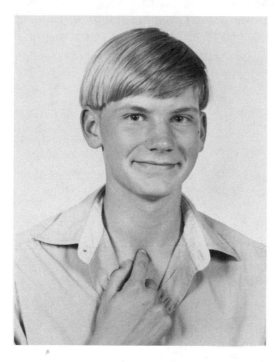

Photo 60: Position for massaging reflexes to the bronchial tubes.

These are reflex buttons on the spine that usually bring almost instant relief to an attack of asthma. It will be helpful if you have another person do the massage for you.

Study Diagram 18B. If you are alone, back up to the edge of a door frame and press the edge into the back as hard as you are able to. The spots will be very tender, but the attack will stop as if by magic as soon as you press on them.

If someone is there to help, either sit or lie face down on a couch or bed, or even on the floor, and have the person press on these spots with the thumb or finger. More than one finger may be used here if the added strength is needed, but it must be centered on the one spot. When another person is pressing on these reflex buttons, then opposites should be pressed simultaneously.

When you find the correct buttons, which will be tender, press firmly and hold for a count of seven. I have seen this stop a bad attack of asthma instantly.

Now massage fairly hard toward the spine. Remember, these reflex buttons are not on the spine, but on the sides of the spine. Notice how #2 spreads lightly away from the spine and #3 spreads still farther toward the shoulder blades. If you have a reflex bar you may be able to use this successfully on yourself.

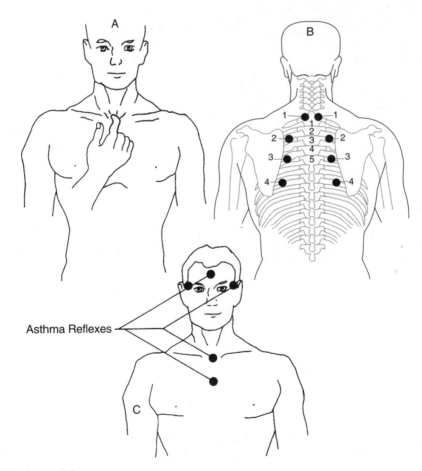

Diagram 18

Immediate Relief from Asthma Attack

Dear Mrs. Carter,

I had been a sufferer from asthma for several years. I had taken all the tests for allergies, but the doctors could find nothing that I was allergic to, except cigarette smoke, so I avoided that. Nothing seemed to help. My husband wanted me to go to a reflexologist. After several more months of suffering and having to go to the hospital and be under oxygen, I decided to take his advice. I went to a professional reflexologist, who was one of your students.

She found certain spots in my body that relieved the coughing and gasping spells immediately. As soon as she touched certain reflexes on my back just below my shoulders and two inches below the neck simultaneously, the asthma attack subsided immediately.

She had decided that the adrenals were affected, and as she worked on the adrenal reflexes, the asthma attacks subsided.

Today, I have very few attacks. If I feel one coming on, I rush to my professional reflexologist to get immediate relief.

—J.M.

REFLEXES TO THE ADRENAL GLAND

The adrenal gland is the culprit that needs special attention when one is suffering from asthma.

In Diagram 2, see that the reflexes to the adrenal gland are located almost in the center of the hand and the foot. Massage these a few moments, and move to the top of the foot and the back of the hand. Press and search for a tender spot above the little finger and above the little toe toward the ankle.

Take the big toe between the thumb and forefinger and press. Search out a tender spot here, and hold or massage for a few moments. You may also do this to the thumb.

Asthma in a Child

I once had a child come to me suffering from asthma, which she claimed to have had since she was very young. No one knew what to do to relieve her.

I started on her feet and worked on all the reflexes that had any connection with asthma. I worked on all the endocrine gland reflexes, which must always be done in any malfunction of the body, no matter what it is. See Diagram 2.

Remember, if just one of the endocrine glands is not functioning perfectly, this causes all the endocrine glands to go out of tune and puts the whole body out of harmony.

I massaged all the body reflexes that I have given you here so that we could stop the asthma and build up lasting protection against further attacks. I taught her how to massage these reflex buttons when she felt an attack coming on and told her to eat honey and to chew the honeycomb. In a short time she was completely free from all signs of asthma, and to this day she is a healthy happy woman with children of her own. She says she keeps her children healthy by using the miracle of reflexology on them when needed.

ADDITIONAL HELP FOR ASTHMATICS

When people have asthma, the upper part of their lungs shows a lack of blood. Turning the patient upside down to allow blood to circulate into the upper part of the lungs relieves the patient considerably. Several helpful positions can bring the asthma sufferer relief. The most important is the yoga headstand. This may be difficult to do for many. There is a device now on the market that will enable anyone to stand on the head comfortably for a long period of time. It is called the "Body Life." Slant boards also help to reverse the pull of gravity on the entire body, increasing blood circulation to all parts of the body from the head to the feet. Another way to get the blood circulating to the upper part of the lungs for quick relief is to lie across the bed on the stomach with the head resting on the hands or arms on the floor.

REFLEXOLOGY HELPS EMPHYSEMA

Use the same reflex buttons for emphysema as you used for asthma, concentrating on the endocrine gland reflexes.

I know a doctor who actually cured many patients of emphysema, some of whom were already bedridden and in their seventies. He had them ride bicycles. First, he put stationary bicycles by their beds and had them start very slowly with just a few strokes at first. As their strength increased, he increased the time they were allowed on the bikes until they were able to ride real bikes outside. He tells us that some of these patients recovered enough to return to work. The motion of riding a bike seems to cause a different way of breathing that is beneficial to the area in which the emphysema is located.

Don't overlook the benefits of the "rebounder." It is like a small trampoline that will fit in any room. This simple little exerciser makes it possible for us to use the three forces of nature—gravity, acceleration, and deceleration. Taking advantage of these forces, we can aid our bodies to overcome many ailments including emphysema. It could even help a smoker to give up smoking.

MUSIC HELPS THE BREATH

I would like to interest you in music. You think this is not the place to talk about music? I think it is. There is a little instrument that you can hold in the palm of your hand that makes beautiful music and can be played by anyone. And it will help build up your breathing power while you are having fun playing your favorite songs. The instrument is the harmonica. Surprised? Just try to blow one a few minutes to see how much wind it takes. If you practice making music or even just a pleasant noise for several minutes a day, you will find that your lungs become more powerful and you can play louder and longer. Start out with a small harmonica and work up to the double reeds later, since these take more wind power than the smaller single-reed ones do. Don't get a cheap harmonica. They are not very expensive, so start with the best. I prefer a "Marine Band." These come in several keys. It will be best to start with the key of C unless you are familiar with music. Books are available to teach you how to play many songs.

All these devices will be beneficial to anyone with lung weakness along with using the reflex massage on all the reflex buttons I have described earlier.

If you really want to get back your breathing power so you can take a deep breath and feel the oxygen surging through your whole body, take the key I have given you, and open the door to a new life.

Daughter Saves Mom from Asthma Attack

A friend of mine told me of a time she and her daughter took an airplane trip across the country, and while they were in flight, she started having an asthma attack. (This attack may have been caused by emphysema.) Amy told me that she grabbed at her chest and tried to catch her breath. Her mouth and throat became dry and she started to panic.

Amy's daughter grabbed her mother's hand and started pressing with her thumbs into the palm; first one hand and then the other, back and forth, about three times. Amy caught her breath and started breathing normally again. Describing her first experience with reflexology, Amy said, "It is very frightening not being able to breathe, especially when you are hundreds of miles up in the sky, with no medication or doctor on board. But my daughter saved me from that fear. I will always love her and am thankful for her fast-acting technique of reflexology."

Ten-Year-Old Girl Saved from Asthma Attack

Dear Mrs. Carter,

I feel everybody should know something about reflexology because they never know when they are going to run into someone who needs help immediately. I met a mother in town the other day who had a ten-year-old girl who was having a bad spell with asthma. The mother was going to drive fifteen miles to the hospital. I told her that the girl needed help immediately because she was about to stop breathing. I showed the mother how to place her center finger in the girl's neck and press in and pull down, and in four seconds she was breathing much better. The little girl told me she didn't think she would have lasted long enough to ride to the hospital. I had a copy of your book in my car, and I showed them Diagram 18 so they would know what to do if the child had another attack.

—E.J.

CHAPTER 28

Relief from Cystic Fibrosis and Multiple Sclerosis

Nutrition Health Review has provided us with new information on the cause and the treatment of one of the terrible degenerative diseases, cystic fibrosis. For more than forty years, the prevailing theory for the cause was that it was a simple "Mendelian genetically transmitted disease." More than $82 million has been devoted to chasing this elusive genetic disease.

According to Merck's *Manual*, there is no cure for the disease. A recommendation is pancreatic enzyme tablets to be taken with each meal with the addition of vitamins A and E.

Veterinarian Discovers the Importance of Selenium

Dr. J. D. Wallach, a veterinarian, was asked to perform an autopsy on a zoo monkey who had died from unknown causes. The examination revealed that the animal had died from cystic fibrosis. Dr. Wallach also discovered that the animal was suffering from a nutritional deficiency—a lack of the mineral selenium.

Dr. Wallach tells us, "Cystic fibrosis, in my opinion, is preventable when caught early enough and is often reversible. The key is a properly balanced diet with adequate selenium supplementation."

Clues for the management of cystic fibrosis were evident as far back as 1951. "In the field of veterinary medicine, there is no lack of knowledge or enthusiasm for proper nutrition. We are very much aware of the importance of minerals in the diet of animals."

If only humans were lucky enough to have the same nutritional management.

HOW REFLEXOLOGY HELPS CONTROL CYSTIC FIBROSIS

Now let us turn to reflexology to help cystic fibrosis. Since the medication that is recommended at this time is mainly pancreatic enzyme replacement, let us concentrate on the reflexes to the pancreas. Refer back to Diagram 2, and find where the pancreas is located in the body. Also, see Diagram 12 and find the reflex to the pancreas on the head. All these reflexes should be stimulated by using pressure with the fingers on these points. Press on these buttons lightly for three seconds, then release. Do this three times to each reflex button. Test for tenderness in the whole area.

While you have the chart to the endocrine glands, stimulate every reflex to these glands. Also, work *every* reflex in the body. Search for "ouch spots" and work them out. You *must* get the healing electrical life force flowing freely to every organ and gland in the body by opening up clogged electrical life lines. Let us prove Dr. Wallach right when he says cystic fibrosis is preventable and even reversible. With proper nutrition and the sensational healing power of reflexology, I believe any ailment can be *prevented* and *cured*.

HELP FOR MULTIPLE SCLEROSIS

If cystic fibrosis can be prevented and cured with nutrition, then, it stands to reason that the same could be true for multiple sclerosis. Many cases of MS have been helped with reflexology. I have seen one woman walk normally within a couple of hours after one treatment on her hands and feet. Now that we are learning more of the reflexes on the body, let us discover even greater health by pressing these magical buttons to open up the free flow of cosmic energy through the electrical lines to all areas of the body. Since we are not sure which glands or organs might be malfunctioning, stimulate *all* of them, concentrating on the reflexes to the brain and spine. Give special attention to the powerful and all-important endocrine gland reflexes, along with a renewed interest in the diet. Reflexology can double your chances of full recovery when used with the correct diet.

Research indicates that MS affects those who may have a weak immune system. If exposed to a virus, a weak immune system will not be able to protect the body from foreign matters or infectious agents. So we must keep the immune system healthy by working the reflexes to revitalize the lymph glands. Work around the wrists, or over the tops of the feet, from ankle to ankle. Repeat several times. As the lymph glands are stimulated, more fluid is circulated to naturally help the body fight off infections and foreign matter. Also work the solar plexus, brain and spine reflex. See Diagrams 3 and 5. Press and hold these reflex buttons to help relax muscles and ease muscle spasms.

Evidence seems to indicate that this crippling disease is caused by malnutrition and is the result of a "civilized" way of life. Most research on the relationship between nutrition and multiple sclerosis has been done in Germany.

Researchers have found that the so-called "primitive" people, for example, Eskimos and some tribes in Africa and Central America, do not contract MS. However, as soon as the Eskimos started to eat "white man's" devitalized and processed food, they contracted the disease in the same proportion as civilized man. There is a firm conviction by some that MS is a degenerative disease caused by an unnatural, unbalanced diet of devitalized foods. Consequently, all experimental treatments in Europe are centering around a nutritional approach.

In the late Paavo O. Airola's book, *Health Secrets from Europe* (Parker Publishing Company), he tells us of Dr. Jorgen Clausen, a Danish biochemist, and his discovery of the deficiency of unsaturated fatty acids and vitamin F in the diet of victims of MS. He also tells us of other European doctors and the successful results they are having in treating multiple sclerosis with nutritional therapy. Two Austrian doctors, Drs. Eckel and Lutz, reported complete or nearly complete recovery by prescribing for their patients a restricted special diet. While this did not affect the more advanced cases, by using reflexology along with this special diet, it may be possible that even the advanced cases could improve.

Many special diets consist of natural foods, such as raw vegetables and fruits, sprouted grains, yeast, and wheat germ. Pure granular lecithin is also very beneficial to one's diet. See Danger of Lecithin, page 119. The myelin sheath, which is the protective covering over the nerves, needs this nutrient. Lecithin helps the system digest, absorb, and carry certain needed vitamins (vitamins A, D, E, and K) in the blood fats and is essential to the cells. The correct diet, coupled with the proper use of reflexology, may, in fact, save a life.

A fellow reflexologist wrote to tell me about her thrilling results after using reflexology. Here is her letter:

> Dear Mrs. Carter,
>
> A friend of mine who has multiple sclerosis was happy to let me give her a reflex treatment. Her right leg had become numb, forcing her to use a cane to walk. During her first treatment, she was able to move her toes, something she hadn't been able to do for a long time. Needless to say, I was thrilled to see what reflexology could do in such a short time.
>
> Yours truly,
>
> —M.A.

Reflex Energy Bypasses Damaged Nerve Fibers

B. F. Hart, M.D., an acupuncture specialist, and physician theorizes that acupuncture may stimulate alternative pathways in the central nervous system in which the message that travels to the body parts actually bypass the nerve fibers that have deteriorated or have damaged portions of the myelin sheath. When using reflexology, the electrical life force moves from the reflex points along the meridians at their own distinction, thus bypassing any damaged nerve fibers. Improved blood supply aids unimpaired nerve functioning while healing forces can promote cellular regeneration.

Dr. Kaslow, acupuncture doctor, tells us that the combination of a diet consisting of unprocessed natural foods and acupuncture to the ear has reduced some crippling effects. One of his patients with MS threw away his cane after only ten treatments! Another student wrote to tell me of the good results he was having with the use of reflexology. Here is the note:

Man Could Feel Tingling in His Feet and Toes

Dear Mrs. Carter,

A man who was visiting family here came to me for help with a blockage of nerves in his leg. His leg and foot became completely numb, and he had *no* feeling at all in them. After just two reflexology treatments, he began to feel tingling in his feet and toes. The improvement was amazing! I know that additional treatments will even help more.

—S.N.R.

Stimulate Electrical Energy to the Brain

A person with MS can self-administer reflexology. By stimulating the nerve endings with a press-and-release motion, voluntary control to affected parts of the body may return. Reflex points on the ears are very easy to work by using a press-and-pinch technique. Work over the entire ear to stimulate every healing reflex. Also give *all* toes and fingers a good workout, especially the tips of big toes and thumbs. This will send electrical life energy to the brain.

Rub your hands together. Now hold the palm of your right hand over the top of the head to generate strength and positive energy. Tapping the top of your head with the middle three fingers of the right hand will stimulate reflexes for healing. Press or tap the reflexes over the cerebral points, and along the longitudinal fissure that runs from the forehead back to the neck. See Diagram 14. This is where the brain is divided into right and left hemispheres. You can also tap over the top of the head from one ear to the other. This is where the motor cortex is located in the brain, and it controls your body's voluntary muscles. This stimulation will be very effective.

Next, place both hands on top of your head, and with very loose fingers, alternate and tap them all at once (as though you are typing very fast). Work with both hands over the cerebral points, along the longitudinal fissure, and then from ear to ear...following the same path as above. (Remember, also, to open up electrical lines to the brain by working the reflexes on the toes and fingers.)

Each individual nerve cell within the brain makes many cell-to-cell connections. As one cell receives information from another, it decides whether to convey the message or not. The decision will depend on the amount of "electrical charge" that the brain cell has on its surface. If it has enough electrical charge, the communication will then be carried across a gap electrically (or by way of molecules—or neurotransmitters); thus, the message will then be transmitted.

Dedicate some serious time to using reflexology, along with a renewed interest in a nutritious diet, and you will be doubling the chances of renewed health.

CHAPTER 29

Using Reflexology to Dissolve Stress and Tension

Stress and anger often cause extreme tension in the body, which tends to make us age sooner and become physically ill and emotionally upset easily. Reflexology gives you the feeling of well-being and calmness, as it helps to normalize your system, creating better circulation and restoring the body to full efficiency.

After using reflexology you will notice all the stress and tensions leaving your body, and as they leave, your mind will also become relaxed. Others may notice how your disposition improves, and you will notice that your responsibilities are easier to approach. As tension gives way to a peaceful, more relaxed attitude, you will soon notice a more positive personality and share a loving disposition with those around you.

Now and then, we all find that we are challenged emotionally or physically. When this happens, we may feel angry, frustrated, or discouraged, as it may seem that we have no control over the difficult situations we encounter. However, with the use of reflexology, we can channel that distressed feeling into a positive force. We must learn to build up our energy and get rid of stress. In just a few words, I am going to show you some very positive ways to accomplish this. You must learn to relax to be healthy, young, and happy.

No matter where you are, you can tap your chest and smile a very big smile to stimulate the thymus gland and lymphatic system.

See Photo 1. The movement of bending your wrist while tapping your chest will pump your lymph fluids. While smiling and tapping your chest, you will be sending renewed energy to your thymus. Your thymus and lymph glands help by changing proteins in your blood into sugar for instant energy.

One day, when I lived in Hawaii, I felt the need to reflex my thymus gland. I was walking down the street in the small town of Kona when I noticed how friendly everyone seemed. People walking by would turn around to give me a nice warm smile and say "hello." Others driving by in their cars would wave to me with beautiful smiles on their faces and shout "Aloha." I was thinking how nice it was to see everyone so happy and carefree that day. Then I remembered…I was exercising the reflex to my thymus gland…and was smiling a big smile from cheek to cheek.

HOW THE ENDOCRINE GLANDS CONTROL STRESS

When you are under stress, it puts a strain on your whole body. Some doctors deem stress the number one killer. It depletes your energy, absorbs nutrients from your system, and creates a hormone imbalance. To build up and restore your hormones to normal, you will need to stimulate the endocrine glands.

Learn the location of reflexes to these glands, as they are *all* important in the health and well-being of every person. Work the reflexes on both feet or both hands to energize this important system. See Diagram 2. These glands are all closely interrelated and supplement and depend on each other for balanced health.

They influence pleasurable emotions such as joy, happiness, excitement, and passion, as well as emotions associated with trauma such as grief, fear, anger, depression, and sadness. Our entire personality and mental outlook depends on the health of the endocrine glands.

Work the big toe or thumb to send energy to the brain and pituitary gland. Our brain is continuously generating electrical currents that are very important to our mental health. Although these currents are not as strong as those that pulse through the heart, they are very important in regulating our emotional well-being.

Give special attention to the thyroid reflex to control your body temperature and calm down that uptight feeling. Then work the reflex to the pancreas, which produces insulin, so that your muscles can convert sugar into energy.

Let us now turn to the adrenals, as they produce adrenalin for extra energy when needed in a hurry. Go to the reflex button on the inside of the hand. The button will be found almost in the center of your palm, on each hand, and up toward the fingers. When you work this reflex, you will also be working the reflex to the solar plexus, which will add to the relaxation of your nervous system and whole body. When you work these reflex buttons you will be awakening some very important elements to physical and mental health. As the vital life force discharges from the endocrine glands, you will become more efficient in your daily work and have a more positive outlook.

NATURE'S METHOD FOR STRESS RELIEF

Have you ever noticed how some people will "wring their hands" when they get nervous? This is a very natural method of stress relief. The fingers of one hand are pressing and stimulating nature's relaxing buttons on the other hand. As one hand rolls inside the other, knuckles are pressing the reflex to the solar plexus and other reflexes, which will relax the whole body.

Another exercise for calming nerves is to clasp both hands together, with fingers intertwined, pressing all the reflexes between fingers seven times. This should relax you considerably. If you are feeling extremely stressed, you can take this exercise a step farther by keeping fingers interlocked, loosening them and moving each finger up over the middle knuckles, squeezing and releasing seven times. Now press the tips of all fingers together with a press-and-release movement. Close your eyes and breathe deeply. As you inhale, you will squeeze your hands together, pressing the reflexes; as you exhale, relax the squeeze and your whole body. Repeat exercise as needed.

WHY DEEP BREATHING IS IMPORTANT FOR CONTROLLING STRESS

Deep, relaxed breathing is one of the most important skills in managing stress and improving mental health. Do you know that your brain uses about one-third of the oxygen you breathe? The air we breathe coordinates with all our movements and mental actions to help us work, play, and think more efficiently.

When one feels stressed, it is common to take short, shallow breaths; however, this will keep your body and mind rigid and uptight. Take a few slow, deep breaths to relax your breathing and calm yourself. Think happy thoughts, and soon your mind will be at rest. You will be surprised how easy this is if you mentally focus on your breathing. As your breathing and thoughts relax, so will your whole body. Soon you will feel free of stress as the tensions naturally fade away.

USE VISUALIZATION FOR RELIEF
FROM ANXIETY

Reflexology is one of the most wonderful, natural methods of relaxing in the world! While you work the reflexes on your body, calm yourself with pleasant and peaceful thoughts. You may enjoy visualizing yourself in another place, somewhere that you would love to be. Imagine the sounds of the seashore, and picture the moon on the beach, listen to each wave as it rolls upon the sand, listen for the seagulls, hear the horn of a boat in the distance. Another time you might like to visualize yourself near a lake, with tall mountains nearby. Listen to the soft breeze in the tall pine trees and hear the tranquility of the birds as they sing their songs of joy. Breathe rhythmically, softly working the reflexes on your feet, hands, head, or ears. Gently work the magical reflex buttons, and soon all tensions will disappear.

Your attitude makes a great difference in your health. Calm your body and stimulate your mind with the healing forces of nature. Give someone you care about a reflex workout or a magic massage ball. See Photo 48. Show them this press-and-go method, and soon you will notice less tension and see a great improvement in their disposition, which will help *you* feel rewarded and less stressed.

RELAX NERVES, NECK, AND SPINE
TO RELIEVE STRESS

First turn to the reflex button at the back of your head called the medulla oblongata. This is where the spinal cord meets the lowest part of the brain. It contains vital nerve centers for controlling your breathing, circulation, and other vital functions. When this reflex is stimulated, it sends energy into your whole being and brings the benefits of relaxation when needed.

Place the middle finger of the right hand into the hollow recess at the back of the head just below the skull. See Diagram 13. Hold for the slow count of three and release; then repeat this several more times. If you move your head forward and backward, you will be able to feel the movement of the top of the spine.

When under stress or tension, we seem to tighten up our muscles which can cause a stiff or sore back. When this happens, work the reflex points to the spine, as well as all the reflexes to the muscles and ligaments connected to the spine. Start working on the reflex to your neck, which can be found around the big toe (or thumb). You can twist the toe (or thumb) around, as you would twist your head, then turn it from side to side. Now work the whole spine reflex. Work up the longitudinal arch of the foot (or down the metacarpel on the hand), pressing with a circular motion to loosen up stiffness.

Work the reflexes to your shoulders and hips on the outside of your feet (or hands). Now look at Diagram 4, and see where the sciatic nerve reflex is on the bottom of the foot and how it travels up the leg. Work the reflex on the bottom of the foot, then work up and down the cords on the back of the legs. The sciatic nerve is a multiple of nerve roots from the lumbar spine. It sends signals down the leg to control muscles and up the leg to stimulate sensations. All these reflexes need attention to completely relax a stiff and sore back. Always remember to work both feet (or hands).

Another method of relaxing tension in the neck is to shrug your shoulders. Pull your shoulders up to your ears, then back down; repeat four or five times. Next, shrug your shoulders up to your ears, then push them backward, as though you were trying to squeeze an orange between your shoulder blades. Relax and repeat four or five times.

Now shake your hands vigorously from the wrists back and forth, as though you were trying to shake water from them. This will promote circulation and release tension. Shake them for about fifteen seconds.

REFLEXOLOGY IS NATURE'S TRANQUILIZER

Reflexology is a natural tranquilizer. Take the time to give yourself a complete reflexology workout, so that nature will move in and relax your entire system. If you are not already familiar with working the reflexes in the feet and hands, I suggest you study the charts. Make sure you are comfortable. Choose a time when you will not be interrupted.

Use a comfortable pressure, yet one that will bring you relief from distress, and then you can enjoy nature's way of relaxing.

Reflexology Worked Better than Tranquilizer

My daughter worked with a man who started experiencing periodic heartburn and stomachaches due to a lot of pressure at work. The pains increased each day until he agreed to see a physician. The doctor diagnosed him by saying, "You are under a great amount of stress, and will soon have stomach ulcers unless you calm down." Tranquilizers were prescribed, and they not only made Jon very tired, but the stress continued. About one hour after Jon took his tranquilizer, he became very sleepy. At work he felt even greater stress because he didn't have the energy needed to complete his job effectively.

One evening after dinner, Jon's wife gave him a complete reflexology workout to promote relaxation. He slept very well that night and seemed to accomplish more at work the following day. And after just one week, he felt such an improvement that he stopped taking the tranquilizers and no longer suffers from heartburn or stomach problems caused from stress. He told my daughter that he is now using "nature's drug-free tranquilizer—reflexology!"

Stimulate Digestion

Some stomach problems, including ulcers, are caused by acids that remain in the stomach and start to burn the stomach walls when you are under stress. This is sometimes called a "nervous stomach."

There is one special reflex point you can work for fast pain relief if you are at work or someplace where you are unable to have a complete reflex workout. This is the web between the index finger and thumb on each hand. Locate the soft spongy spot about an inch into the triangle, squeeze and rotate with a press-and-pinch technique to stimulate the proper functioning of your digestive system. See Photo "C." Also work the pad below the thumb. See Photo "D."

Reach up and give your ears a good rub from time to time, and bring them a vigorous, flourishing supply of blood. See Photos 19 and 20. Soon your body and nerves will all be totally relaxed.

Remember that a simple finger exercise is great for releasing tensions. Start with a tight fist, open each finger, starting with the little one until all fingers are opened up wide. Repeat four times, rub hands together, and then slightly shake to release stress.

Another of nature's natural-stress release methods is simply to yawn and stretch. You can feel the tensions disappear.

Slow Down Your Heart Rate

If you find yourself in a stressful situation and your heart starts pounding very fast and hard, you need to stop what you are doing and take a rest. Don't let stress or anger get out of control; a reflex workout will calm you down. Work the reflex points to your heart, which you will find on your left hand (and your left foot). Work all the way across the palm and down around the little finger. This will help you regain your calm as you send healing forces to your heart. See Diagrams 3 and 5.

Another quick method to slow down a furiously beating heart rate is one that I learned from a man in Arizona. Place your left hand, including pulse area at wrist, into some icy cold water. (Use both hands or dip your feet if you prefer.) You may also splash some on your face and all around your neck. As your blood cools, your heart rate will slow down. Researchers have learned from studying dolphins that as they go into icy water, their hearts slow down. This holds true for us, too.

15 Ways to Alleviate Stress and Tension

1. Give yourself a nice hand and foot rub. Reflexology is the key to complete relaxation.
2. Elevate your feet and clear your mind of negative thoughts.
3. Wear comfortable shoes and go for a nice brisk walk.
4. Close your eyes and visualize an enjoyable experience, pleasurable sensation or relaxing location.
5. Take time to enjoy working on a favorite hobby.
6. Participate in a sport or activity that you enjoy.
7. Talk to a friend with a good sense of humor. Laughter reduces anxiety.
8. Take several deep breaths and breathe naturally.
9. Water is very relaxing. Sit by a stream or take a swim.
10. Do some simple stretching exercises to reduce tense muscles and joints.

11. Have a massage.

12. Get proper rest and give nature the opportunity to restore and renew your body.

13. Eat a well balanced diet from the four food groups and drink plenty of water.

14. Read, do crossword puzzles or play cards.

15. Pressure points between fingers will calm you. Fold your hands together and clasp tightly (repeat seven times). Shake hands. Breathe deeply and relax!

How to Revitalize Your Physical Energy to Reduce Stress

Stress depletes your energy—when your body has no mental or physical power for action, you need to revitalize yourself with a reflex workout. First, give an energetic workout to *all* of your reflexes for fast, renewed energy. Do not miss the liver reflex, as it may need stimulation to filter out harmful properties that make you feel sluggish.

Do this by first sitting down, then reaching down with both hands and taking hold of one foot. Place your fingers on the sole of your foot and your thumbs on top. See Photo "G." Press down and out with the heel and thumb of both hands. At the same time press into the bottoms of your feet with your fingers. Using a press-and-pinch method, work fast to get the circulation moving.

Give your feet a fast vigorous rub, pressing on several reflexes at once. Press on the bones beneath the skin, and with firm movements work your hands quickly over and under your feet and toes. Then work around to the back of your foot, and up the leg a bit with a squeezing motion. Repeat on other foot. You will feel a boost of energy, and stress will soon disappear.

Reflexology for Seniors and Children

I enjoy teaching reflex points to seniors and little children. When visiting nursing homes and classrooms, I find that they like learning new ways to help themselves feel better. One reflex they especially like is the one to their solar plexus (a network of nerves in the abdominal cavity that sends nerve impulses to the upper middle part of the abdomen). When this reflex is stimulated, it relaxes the whole system.

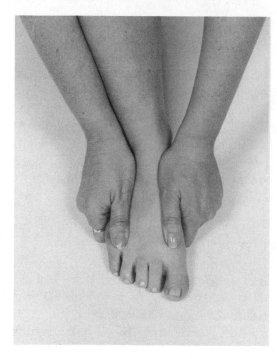

Photo "G": Work reflexes vigorously for renewed energy. Also important reflex to Lymphatic System, helps defend body against disease.

The solar plexus reflex is easy and fun to find. Take one of your hands and make a tight fist, now look into the fist and find where your middle finger and ring finger meet the palm. Between the tip of these two fingers is where we find the reflex button. Press it with the thumb of your opposite hand, count to three very slowly, take a deep breath, and then gently release the pressure. Repeat six times, and the stress or anger will go away.

People can learn to calm themselves when they get angry or upset with someone—and it makes them feel a little more secure. One youngster, about six years old, told me, "When I get mad at my brother, I push my 'solar button' and feel nice."

CONTROL STRESS AND ANGER WITH LAUGHTER

We talked about how good it is for everyone to smile. Now let me explain the health benefits of laughter. A good hearty laugh will calm various emotional disturbances. Anxiety and tension will be released very quickly after a good laugh, because as a person laughs, chemicals in the brain are elevated, thus reducing depression and anxiety. Laughter is a tranquilizer with no side effects. Laughter is a powerful, healing force.

Studies have been done at the University of California, in Davis, to see if laughter plays an active role in protecting one's health. The studies show that laughter is great for the lungs and respiratory system and is a great workout for all internal organs. Several good hearty laughs a day are equal to five minutes of rowing a boat.

You will be surprised at how laughter will rejuvenate you both mentally and physically, as well as help dissolve built-up hostility or anger. So go ahead laugh, and feel the stress fade away.

USE REFLEXOLOGY FOR RESTFUL SLEEP

Do you squeeze your eyes closed when you are sleepy? If so, you are naturally pressing nature's "sleep buttons." These little reflex points can be found just above the inside corner of each eye.

Press inward and upward here, using the tips of your thumbs (the knuckles of index fingers work well for those with long fingernails). Or use your thumb and index finger to squeeze the bridge of your nose between your eyes. Squeeze and hold for fifteen seconds. Repeat several times.

Reflex Ears, Neck, and Hands for Fast Sleep

A friend of mine discovered a natural, creative technique that produces such a calm state of relaxation that she usually falls asleep before she is finished with the exercise.

First, she uses the yawn and stretch exercise that is found on page 235 of my *Hand Reflexology* book. Then she places her hands on her ears, and thoroughly works all the reflexes for about thirty seconds. She then moves to the neck and works down the tendons. Working one side at a time, she presses and rubs all the way down her left arm into her hand, then gives her hand a good workout. Next, she repeats on the right side. She ends by using reflexology to overcome insomnia, found on page 261 of this book. She also pays attention to her breathing, keeping it rhythmic, and claims this works every time.

Use the Foot Massager for Restful Sleep

I like to use the type of foot massager that you put on the floor and roll under the feet. This stimulates most of the reflexes to the whole body. You will become so totally relaxed, you may fall to sleep in the chair. All your glands and organs will function naturally and without tensions or stress, when your body is calm and relaxed.

While you sleep, your body is rebuilding new cells and tissues. This is the best time for healing.

Prevent the Cause of Your Sleep Loss

Breathe slowly and deeply and use reflexology to calm and relax your whole body for a wonderful tense-free sleep. If you are bothered by something that is preventing you from getting your much needed sleep, consider the immediate environment. If you are losing sleep from bright lights, wear an eye mask. If a noise is keeping you awake, use earplugs. Bad weather? If it's too cold, wear long johns, or if it's too hot, place a cool damp cloth under your feet and hands and turn on a fan. Sleep may not come easily if you have consumed caffeine late in the day. A good rule to follow is never to drink or eat a stimulant after 4:00 P.M. If you are kept from your much needed sleep because of illness, use reflexology to relax and calm you down. You will soon be happily resting.

Reflexology Helps Overcome Insomnia

If you feel tired, but just can't seem to drift off to sleep, try this exercise. Lay on your back, hands clasped over your chest. Press and release your interlocked fingers together seven times, putting the pressure between each finger close to the hand. Keeping fingers interlocked, loosen them and move each finger up over the knuckles, with a press-and-release movement. Close your eyes and breathe deeply. As you inhale, squeeze your hands together, pressing the reflexes between each finger. As you exhale, relax the squeeze and your whole body. Repeat the exercise.

One very simple reflex point to clear your tension and enable you to sleep is located on each side of your forehead, just at the outer end of each eyebrow. Use tips of index fingers, or your knuckles, and work these reflexes simultaneously for fifteen seconds. Release and repeat for three to four minutes. See Photo "F."

Foods That Help You Sleep

Foods make changes in the body, as well as in the brain and may affect your sleep. Milk products, such as cottage cheese, may invite sleep. Warm milk with a banana or a piece of bread has been known to increase drowsiness. The amino acids from the food goes into the bloodstream, which in turn travels to the brain and lets it know that you are tired. One recipe that has worked for many is to warm one cup of pure water and add two tablespoons pure honey and one tablespoon *either* apple cider vinegar *or* fresh lemon juice. Sip this very slowly. Afterward, brush your teeth well to remove all honey and vinegar. Now off to bed, and have sweet dreams!

Mentally Focus on Your Breathing

If you are feeling stressed, you need to mentally focus on how you are breathing. Take a few slow, deep breaths to help you relax. Think happy thoughts, and soon you will be able to rest your mind. As your breathing and thoughts relax, so will your whole body. Soon your tensions will fade away, and you will feel wonderfully at ease. Press the reflex to your solar plexus in the center of your hand to relax your nerves.

When Physical Disorders Cause Loss of Sleep

When you're in pain, your body is tense, and it is hard to have a peaceful sleep. When you are tense, your muscles contract, causing the natural flow of blood to be constricted. (If there is swelling, more circulation would be cut off.) It is very important to circulate the flow of blood to any afflicted areas within your body to relieve distress. Working the appropriate reflex points on your hands to relieve pain will be helpful. See Photo "C."

With the use of reflexology, your body will relax and circulation will improve. Healing will progress faster, and you will soon enjoy your much needed slumber without pain.

How to Rid Problems of Elimination

Elimination problem can cause sleep loss. The organs of elimination work around the clock, whether the body is awake or sleeping. You can strengthen these organs by working the reflex buttons to the colon, lungs, kidneys, and bladder so they will flush out wastes.

Stimulate the lymph glands, adrenals, and heart with a good reflex workout, to condition and balance your system so that you will receive the reward you deserve...a peaceful night's sleep.

A Kind Gentle Word Will Move Mountains

Dear Ms. Carter:

God did not make a cheap imitation of any human being. We are all works of art which have the capability of rejuvenating ourselves through stimulation. Most illnesses become physical but basically start mentally through loneliness, stress, environmental pressures, circumstances, learned behavior, etc. . . . And, many times, the power of suggestion that a person can be healed is more powerful than any medication they could take. You see, medication dulls the sensation, but a loving stroke and a kind, gentle word will move mountains; it renews a person's importance in life and shows them that they are somebody and worthy of love.

I have learned we can calm nerves and stress. Since sebaceous glands become over stimulated in times of stress, this often causes acne outbreak. A session of reflexology eases the tension and slows the oil activity restoring the glands to a normal state. I also realized if I stimulated the energies from the foot, moved to the hands to the ulna and radial nerve in the arms, up to the stress in the neck and shoulder, to the pressure points on the face, ears, scalp and head . . . our friends would become whole new people.

Sincerely,

—B.V.L.

CHAPTER 30

Reflexology Provides an Alternative to Addictions

Reflexology provides a positive alternative to addictions such as drinking, eating, smoking, gambling, sex, taking drugs, and so on, which can all contribute significantly to major health problems. Reflexology can dissolve tension and replace it with a deep relaxation, and a calm soothing feeling. As your system relaxes, reflexology maximizes your body's abilities to heal from within. If someone you know has an addiction, you can help him or her with reflexology.

HELP FOR ALCOHOLISM

Doctors are finding that alcoholism is a glandular disorder that can be compared to diabetes. When a person has diabetes, not enough insulin is produced, resulting in high blood sugar. However, in the case of alcoholics, too much insulin is produced which results in low blood sugar. The two main glands involved are the adrenals and the gland which regulates them, the pituitary. Another very important gland is the pancreas, which produces insulin.

First we must concentrate on the reflex to the pituitary gland, as it controls the other glands. You will find pituitary buttons located in the center of the pad on the bottom of both big toes, and the pad on both thumbs. See Diagram 2.

264

Now we will move on to the reflexes of the adrenal glands and pancreas, still using the hand and foot reflexes. Place your thumb on the reflex area of the kidney, and work the thumb up just a little toward the fingers, (or toes) and you will be on the reflex to the adrenal gland. Work this area with a press-and-roll motion.

Look at the diagram to see where the pancreas reflex is located. It is very close to the kidneys and stomach reflex. You can continue to massage almost clear across the hand (or foot). Working the reflex to the liver is very important, and remember if it is tender, only work on the point for a minute, then return to it later. And never forget to work the lymph glands to flush out harmful chemicals and waste materials.

The stimulation to these very important glands and organs will bring the healing life force back into them so that the body will be able to return to normal functioning.

Mr. H. had a problem with drinking all of his life. He wrote to tell me how reflexology has helped him.

Reflexology Helps Alleviate a Drinking Problem of Forty-eight Years

Dear Mrs. Carter,

I have cirrhosis of the liver and have been using your technique for four months. In that time, I haven't had a drink. I started to drink at eighteen and am now sixty-six. This is the first time I have been able to do without it. For the first time in years, I can eat well, and I am feeling really great.

Thank you,

—Mr. F.H.

EAR REFLEX WORKOUT HELPS TREAT WITHDRAWAL SYMPTOMS

One way addicted people can help themselves is to reach up and work the reflexes on the ear. This is especially helpful when someone is feeling stressful from withdrawal symptoms. See Diagram 15. Start at the top of the ear, where the toes and foot reflexes are located. Work this part of the ear for one or two minutes, then work down. Stop at the center of the ear, where the liver and spleen reflex are located. You will want to work this reflex for about two minutes, and then work down to the earlobe. Work the reflexes on the front and back of the lobe with a pressing, pinching motion. Five or ten minutes can be spent on each ear, then relax the pressure. Repeat this as often as needed, or until the person recovers and feels no further need for the treatment.

A reflex clamp can be used to put pressure on the ear lobe (see Photo 18) as pressing with the finger and thumb in this position for any length of time may become tiring. This has been reported as working wonders at alleviating certain addictions. Reflexology methods are used to help recover from hangovers and headaches, as well as calm the frustration, tension, and pain of withdrawal symptoms. Just grab a big handful of hair and pull it upward and outward. Hold it there for 15 seconds, then release. Grab another handful and pull it, continuing this method to stimulate the reflexes in your whole body, including your stomach and internal organs. See Photo 9.

Also, tapping the head with a wire brush is helpful when one is recovering from a hangover. See Photo 11.

REFLEXOLOGY AND DRUGS

Most of the drugs that go into the body will be metabolized in the liver and excreted by way of the kidneys. Therefore, the reflex to these organs, as well as the reflexes to the endocrine glands, should receive extra attention to balance the body and encourage the excretion in the liver. See Diagrams 2, 3 and 5.

You may find that the reflex to the liver and kidneys will be tender, as poisons released from other organs in the body will give them extra work. Reflexology, good nutrition, and exercise will bring healing to the body, determination and confidence to the mind, and guidance to the spirit. Habit control is essential for a happy, long and pain-free life. Again I must remind you how many functions of the body depend on water and air. Proper hydration is critical, and air is essential to all our lives, especially when the body is healing itself from drug abuse. Remember, vitamin C and potassium are vital for flushing poisonous substances from your body.

Employment Drug Test

Dear Mrs. Carter,

I went for a job interview and the company had me take a drug-use urine test. The investigation into my private life was insulting, and since a small amount of a drug was found in my urine, I did not get the job. I went home, studied your book, and gave myself a reflex workout. I really worked the lymph glands, especially at the top of both feet, on the hollow area.

One week later I returned and took the test again, and was found drug-free! I am now on the waiting list for a job. I do not need or want drugs in my life ever again. I always experience a unique serenity and a wonderful feeling of tranquillity after each reflex workout. Thanks to your help, I am now more productive and have far fewer health problems than ever before.

—M.N.

PREVENTING OXYGEN STARVATION FOR SMOKERS

A heavy smoker will suffer from lack of oxygen, which will cause the heart to pump faster than usual in order to get the necessary amount of oxygen. And when the proper amount of oxygen is not taken into the lungs, the brain suffers. Make sure you draw oxygen-filled air down into the very bottom of your lungs so that your body will not suffer from oxygen starvation. Use the deep breathing techniques I described earlier in the book.

HOW TO TEST YOUR LUNG FUNCTION

Get an ordinary match, light it, hold it at arm's length, inhale a deep breath, aim straight and blow out the flame. If this is easy for you, your lungs are most likely functioning well. If you can't blow out the flame, you will need to work the reflex area to the heart and circulatory system, and the respiratory system (mainly the lungs and heart, see Diagrams 3 and 5), and practice your deep breathing. Then try this test again in a few days and you should be able to blow out the match.

SMOKERS, PAST AND PRESENT BENEFIT
FROM REFLEXOLOGY

Smoking changes the blood chemistry, which will cause constrictions in the blood vessels of fingers and toes, causing poor circulation. Reflexology will improve blood circulation throughout your body. One man I know who smokes complained of toe cramps and cold feet. After just two reflex treatments, he said his feet felt warm and he didn't suffer pain in his toes.

Reflexology is also very beneficial after you have stopped smoking as it will help to flush the harmful carcinogens from your system. You will no longer have to worry about a disease or illness that might develop from your previous smoking habit. This reflex stimulation will bring a vigorous new life force to the organs and glands for a healthy body and a happy soul.

REFLEXOLOGY HELPS SOLVENT ABUSERS

Most solvent abusers have difficulty sleeping, are highly stressed, may become anemic, develop chronic kidney inflammation and can suffer liver failure. Therefore, a full reflexology treatment must by given. Attention should be given to all vital organs, with emphasis on the lungs and liver, endocrine glands, brain, and spine. The problem of solvent abuse with substances such as glue, which are sniffed, gas or drugs, is now becoming very widespread. An estimated one in every ten young people will experiment with dangerous solvents. I have heard from teachers who use reflexology to calm many situations, both in secondary schools, and in schools for deprived children. Parents and voluntary reflexologists come to the aid of these students, who often have low self-esteem and struggle with peer pressure. These volunteers take the time to really *listen* to the students and teach them to calm their lives with deep breathing and reflexology. These results are wonderful.

You can help also, by encouraging those affected by solvents or chemicals to drink a lot of water, and show them how to use reflexology to flush toxic wastes from their system. Also, you will want to teach the importance of deep breathing. Refer to Chapter 12.

REFLEXOLOGY AND EXPOSURE TO DANGEROUS CHEMICALS

With a lot of concern for the young people who experiment with solvents, we also worry about the many people who work around solvents, or those who are exposed to chemicals without protection from dangerous fumes. People working in industries without proper ventilation may suffer from similar health problems.

I received a letter from the wife of a Vietnam veteran who would like to see a full staff of reflexologists in every military hospital. Her husband was exposed to Agent Orange, which caused a chemical change in his body. Here is her letter, which tells how they are dealing with this problem:

How Reflexology Helps Vietnam Veteran

Dear Mrs. Carter,

My husband was exposed to Agent Orange in Vietnam. Doctors say the body performs some sort of chemical change so that the Agent Orange is not recognizable in the body in its original form. It is, however, recognizable by its sufferers who are still subject to its effects twenty-plus years later. One of the symptoms is periodic depression.

My husband and I first learned of reflexology about three years ago. Over this time I have accumulated some knowledge from books and from other reflexologists. But for the past ten months, I have been massaging my husband's feet on a regular basis and with a great deal more understanding. We can recognize clearly when that tendency toward depression begins. I will massage his feet immediately and everyday for perhaps three or four days. The feeling of depression vanishes without any episodes of anti-social behavior. The effect of the massage is immediate. He will come in and complain that he feels terrible. He'll plop down in the recliner and I'll start on his feet. When I finish a good vigorous massage, he says he feels better and can think better. He gets up and finishes his day's work. (We live on a ranch which he manages, so he does have some flexibility to do that.)

Reflexology has given us a new life. It is still a constant battle, and I don't know if it is possible for his body to throw off that terrible toxin. But it is obvious that massaging his feet twice a week (and sometimes more) creates a much better state of health in general and seems to raise his level of pain tolerance. (He has a piece of shrapnel in his leg which gives him constant pain.) I would like to see a whole staff of reflexologists in every V.A. and military hospital, and I wish every veteran's wife knew reflexology—not only for her husband's sake, but for her sake as well.

—C.E.

HELP STOP ADDICTIONS BY USING REFLEXOLOGY ON EARS

One way people can help themselves when faced with an unwanted addiction, is to reach up and work the reflexes on their ears. See Diagram 15. Using pressure on the reflexes in the ears will correct many symptoms of habitual inclination. And it is especially helpful when someone is feeling stressful from withdrawal symptoms.

Start at the top of the left ear, using thumb and middle finger, with a pinch-and-roll technique, and work clear across the upper part of the ear for one or two minutes. See Photo 19.

Now work down the ear and stop at the center (where the reflex to the liver and spleen are located). Using the tip of your middle finger, press this reflex point with a very small circular motion for one minute. (This area will probably be very tender.) Continue working on down the ear by pressing and squeezing each reflex to the slow count of seven. Work on down to the ear lobe, stimulating the reflexes, both on the front and back of the ear. See Photo 20. Repeat on the right ear.

Five or ten minutes can be spent on each ear to reduce patients' need for their addiction. These reflex buttons can be used as often as needed to free the addictive behavior. Working with the finger and thumb in this position for any length of time may become tiring; if so, a reflex clamp can be used to put pressure on the ear lobe. See Photo 18.

The healing energy of ear reflex therapy has been reported as working wonders to free the craving of certain addictions. Some subjects reported complete renewal of their health and freedom from their addictions with the use of reflexology. Reflexology is nature's way to deal with distress, and is a wonderful alternative to any addiction!

CHAPTER 31

How Reflexology Helps You Lose Weight Naturally

How would you like to press a button and watch the unwanted fat melt off your body just like magic? You can use reflexology to dissolve those unwanted pounds easily and naturally, just by knowing the location of a few special buttons to press.

Acupuncture doctors have used needles very successfully to help many people lose weight. But you don't need needles or a doctor since you can use the method of reflexology to accomplish the same thing safely in your own home.

Now some of these pressure points that I am going to teach you to use are reflexes that directly affect the hunger cells inside the brain. So, if we press on a key reflex to the part of the brain that affects the appetite, we will trick that particular cell, so that the brain tells your stomach that it is satisfied. (Which means it will not send out a hunger message.) If we use this reflex therapy before meals, we will reduce the pangs of hunger and eat less.

One should never eat unless one is hungry. The stomach is not ready to accept food, and when food is forced into it, the acids cannot work to digest the food properly. Thus, we have an upset stomach of various kinds.

Dr. Bahr has a clinic in Munich for reducing overweight people, and he claims to have successfully reduced over a thousand overweight people in one year with pressure of certain buttons on the face and body. One of the people who lost many pounds with this method was Dr. Bahr himself. He claims that in two months he lost more than thirty pounds. Dr. Bahr claims to have just discovered this wonderful, fantastic method of reducing, and many doctors all over Europe are using it with great success. The doctors claim that the beauty of this method of reducing is that it is absolutely harmless and that the procedure stops unnecessary appetite, but does not affect real hunger.

We who have used reflexology in this country for many years are well aware of the reflex points that will help in not only repressing the appetite, but also in stimulating certain glands and organs to help the body lose unnecessary fat.

How Reflexology Controls the Appetite

I know some of you have tried every method available for losing weight with no success. But now with the help of reflexology, you can at last find yourself buying the smaller sizes that you have always dreamed of wearing, while you become more beautiful and energetic and feel like a million dollars.

How Reflexology Works
for the Overeater

We will first learn how reflexology works for the overeater. One reflex is above the upper lip, and another is in the ear. Let us start with the reflex above the lip. It is just above the center of the lip between the nose and the edge of the lip. Look at Diagram 12 of the head. Notice all the important gland reflexes that are located above the lip, under the nose. Three very important endocrine glands are stimulated here when we press this one area. We know that the pineal and pituitary glands are located in the center of the head, and the pancreas and spleen are also very valuable reflexes. (See Diagram 2, which is the chart of the endocrine glands.) Press on this reflex above the upper lip to open up the electrical force line to the brain, as well as to the pancreas and the spleen to curb those hunger pangs.

(This combination reflex button has many benefits. Here I will list a few of them for you. Pressing it helps with mental alertness and is beneficial to some types of paralysis. Also you can press the side of your index finger up against your nose and on the center of the upper lip reflex button at the same time to stifle a nosebleed and to stop a sneeze.)

One way to find the exact pressure point is to place the index or middle finger, whichever is easier for you, beneath the nose. You will now press with a rotating motion for about ten counts, putting pressure against the upper jaw. Repeat three or four times to help repress the appetite. See Photos 46 and "H." Remember, when you are working these reflexes, they will be more effective when you are centered on the right spot.

HOW TO SUPPRESS THE APPETITE

Now let us go to the ears for further help in suppressing the appetite. A short time ago, it was the fashion to go to an acupuncture doctor to have little needles or staples placed in the ears to stop the pangs of hunger. Every time the person felt hungry, they were to press on these little devices, and they would no longer feel the need for food. And in many cases, it worked. But you don't need to have pins placed in your ears to get the same results. These very same doctors tell us how we can use the fingers to accomplish the same results.

Dr. Robert E. Willner, a physician and acupuncture specialist, tells us that your hunger pangs stop almost immediately if you use this technique of working these reflexes. If you use this reflex massage for a minute or so, your appetite will be gone. According to ancient acupuncture principles, this technique will suppress hunger from one to five hours, and you can use it as often as it is needed.

First, you will insert the tip of your index fingers gently into the ears, palms facing toward the front of your face (toward your cheeks). Now, using the thumb, you will press on the small flap above the earlobe. (See Diagram 15 and notice the reflex buttons to forehead and back of head. The button to repress the appetite, can be found between them.) With the reflex point between the thumb and index finger, you will work with a rolling, squeezing motion for at least one minute. Now using the third finger, you will press on the small indention just in front of the frontal lobe (or tragus) and very slightly above it. You will work these small reflex buttons in a circular motion for at least one minute each.

You can use this method of reflexology to stop hunger before meals, and you will be satisfied eating less. It can also be used at the end of a meal or even during the meal if you feel that you need it. You may use either one of these reflex points, or both.

Dr. Albert Fields, an acupuncture examiner for California's Board of Medical Quality Assurance, tells us these points should be used repeatedly, four to six times a day and before meals. It helps you overcome the temptation of eating between meals and also will help you eat less at your meals.

It is said that massaging these reflexes works on hunger by direct nerve action, as there are five major cranial nerves sending branches to the ear, one of them being the vagus nerve, which is the major nerve involving the digestive system. It affects the secretions and movement of the gastrointestinal system. Thus, when you work these reflexes, they normalize the hunger signals going to the brain—your appetite is normalized, and you will no longer be unnecessarily hungry!

Now that we have learned how to suppress the appetite to enable us to eat less, let us turn to the reflexes that will help the body throw off fat, which it may have accumulated over the years. We will now turn to the reflexes elsewhere in the body to further help dissolve unwanted fat.

Since we have stimulated the reflexes in the face to the pineal, pituitary, spleen, and pancreas, let us give them added stimulation by pressing reflex buttons elsewhere in the body. Look at the chart of the endocrine glands, especially the adrenal and thyroid glands, in the front of the book (Diagram 2), and also the charts showing the liver, colon, and kidneys (Diagrams 3 and 5). You will want to stimulate and work these special reflexes to help the body melt off hard-to-lose fat.

Remember the vital importance of your diet. Make sure you get lots of vitamin C and potassium daily. Vitamin C is necessary for maintaining your body's supply of collagen, which is a protein that forms connective tissue in your bones, ligaments, and skin, and it is vital for flushing out poisonous substances. Together potassium and vitamin C work like cleansing agents to wash out fats and unclog arteries.

By using reflexology, vitamin C and potassium every day you will rid toxic poisons from your system and help fight against cellulite. Your new body will be beautiful and *healthy* naturally, without the use of "diet pills" or any other harmful substances.

REFLEXOLOGY, EXERCISE, AND DIET HELP WEIGHT REDUCTION

When you eat sugar and starch, some of it turns into yellow fat cells, and weight gain will continue as long as these cells build up. So remember the importance of a healthy eating program, and choose only nutritionally balanced foods from the food pyramid. When purchasing foods, read all food labels and stay away from harmful fats, such as coconut and palm oil. When preparing meals, use cooking methods such as steaming, baking, broiling, and grilling rather than frying.

Exercise is another important key to losing weight. The internal organs cannot function well with drooping, sluggish muscles, so tighten up your abdominal structure. Studies show that dieting alone is not as effective as dieting combined with exercise. The reason is that as you decrease your calories, your metabolic rate also decreases. Therefore, unless you get enough exercise, your system will not burn off calories as quickly as it did, and your weight loss will slow down, or completely stop. Walking or a moderate workout after a meal will burn off more fat and calories than if you take your walk on an empty stomach. However, you will want to use low-intensity exercise right after a meal, so that you will not upset your digestive system.

Be determined, apply the power of your mind to your weight-loss program, and you will soon be a lot healthier and will look and feel a lot younger! With the combination of exercise and reflexology, you will lose excess weight, detoxify the body, and control the appetite so that you will be the healthy person you have always wanted to be!

HOW REFLEXOLOGY AND A SECRET METHOD OF EATING WILL BURN OFF AND FLUSH OUT FAT

You may have heard of the "foods that melt fat" from your body. Well, it is true! These are foods such as raw fruits and vegetables. Whichever are in season, and are fresh, will be fine. These raw foods have certain substances that are produced by living cells that act as catalysts that take place within the metabolism to break down and wash out fat before it has a chance to attach to your cells.

The secret is...you must eat a raw food *before and after* your meal. That's right...eat raw foods, such as cabbage, carrots, or cucumbers before your meal. Then after the meal you will want to eat parsley, apple, banana, or another raw food. This way the enzymes are working hard to break down all the fats from that meal. This secret method of eating, coupled with a complete reflexology workout, will cause a metabolic reaction that will burn off and flush out those unwanted calories from your body. Just watch the pounds melt away! You will notice the difference in just one week.

WHY REFLEXOLOGY IS IMPORTANT WHEN DIETING

As you lose weight, your body will be releasing fat, and on its way out, a little may move into the bloodstream. If this happens, a uric acid buildup may cause you to feel like you have indigestion. Reflexology is very beneficial at this time, and will help energize your internal organs and the circulatory, digestive, and urinary systems will all work hard to flush out any accumulated waste.

As extra weight comes off, your whole body will be affected. This is why a complete reflexology workout to all parts of your body is the best method to keep emotionally and physically well. Soon your entire system will be balanced with good health and will be free from excess weight.

Why Water and Fiber Are Important When Dieting

Many studies have shown that when people add more water to their diet, fat deposits are reduced. When people drink less water, fat deposits increase. Tests clearly show us that water washes away the pounds.

Water in the system helps the kidneys function properly; however, if the kidneys do not receive the needed amount of water, then the liver must do their work. We do not want to give this overload to the liver, for then it could not do its own work—the liver's primary function is to metabolize stored fat into energy—so let it do its work. If the body does not have enough water, neither the liver nor the kidneys can metabolize fat.

Most people should drink six eight-ounce glasses of water daily. However, the person who has extra weight has a greater metabolic rate, and needs to drink an additional eight-ounce glass of water for every twenty pounds of excess body weight. Work the reflex to the kidney and to the liver, and drink pure water everyday to help keep the weight off.

Salt will contribute to body retention of water and may add problems of cellulite. You can add one tablespoon of pure apple cider vinegar to one eight-ounce glass of water and drink it with each meal. The vinegar contains potassium, which will break up, and wash out, the fats. Use a straw to drink from, as too much vinegar on your teeth may eat away at the enamel.

Now let's look at the studies done on fiber: These results showed that when people add high fiber to their meals, they are able to lose weight much faster than those who don't get enough fiber.

Fiber will naturally suppress the appetite because it absorbs and holds a great deal of water; therefore, we do not have that hungry feeling so often. Fiber also absorbs excess fats from food and the intestines, so remember when you are using reflexology to give special attention to reflexes of the organs of elimination to help keep the fats and fluids moving out of the body.

The combination of reflexology, water, and fiber is an excellent system to achieve successful weight loss.

How Dieting Can Cause Constipation

When you change your eating habits, your internal organs do not always know how to react to the changes. If you diet, keep in mind to add fiber. If not enough fiber is added to your diet, constipation may result.

One young man who had lost over sixty pounds when he came to see me had been suffering from constipation. We used reflexology to get his system stimulated. First, a complete reflex workout was used on his feet, with added attention given to the small intestine and colon reflex area. We needed to promote some digestive juices to help move bulk and waste matter. Along with the reflex therapy, I gave him a few nutritional tips, which included the use of bran and wheat germ sprinkled on yogurt, or mixed in a glass of juice. I also gave him some herb-lax tea to help break up the bulk. It seems when he went on a diet and started eating small amounts of food, his bowels just stopped functioning, and this caused him severe cramps and constipation.

The following week he called to tell me that the tea, added fiber, and reflexology methods I showed him all worked. He no longer had those terrible cramps, nor did he have constipation, and his weight loss was continuing with rapid success. He was happy to tell me that he felt great!

Healthy elimination is necessary to balance your system when dieting. When this energy is blocked, it will affect not only your weight but your emotions as well.

Remember to never degrade yourself by hanging posters of sumo wrestlers around your kitchen. Instead, focus all your energy on positive thoughts, and be thankful for who you are. Place positive notes where you can see them often. They can say "I am thinner today, I look and feel better than ever!" Your willpower will be much stronger when you give yourself positive encouragement. I am sure you are a beautiful person; remember to accept yourself completely, and each day you will be happier and become more confident.

Shannon's Story

Shannon came to me with a list of many illnesses. She thought she had edema, plus other ailments, and was frightened about what a doctor might tell her. She called me one week before her doctor's appointment. She wanted to see what reflexology could do for her. Shannon was forty-five years old, was 5 feet 7 inches tall, and weighed 237 pounds. She was under a lot of stress at work and felt this was the reason for her overeating.

After a complete reflexology session with Shannon, we realized that all she needed was to lose weight. None of her reflexes were tender, with the exception of her kidneys. She needed to flush some very harmful toxic fluids from her body, so I taught her how to give herself a basic foot reflex workout. It was easy for her to lift her feet, and she liked this method. I also showed her the reflexes to control her appetite on her lip and ear. I gave her a Magic Reflex Massager and told her to use it for one minute on each hand, whenever she got up for a snack. And instead of a snack, she should drink a six-ounce glass of cranapple juice to clear her bladder.

Shannon returned to see me twice. She has been doing well. She lost ten pounds in two weeks and made significant progress in controlling the urge to eat when she felt tension at work. With the use of reflexology, Shannon feels the loss of weight will be gradual, but to her that is okay. She said "even if it takes a few years to reach my goal, I will be happy because reflexology and walking has made it possible for my system to burn off fat, not to store it, or gain any more!" Shannon didn't need to see the doctor, and plans to stay in shape for the rest of her life. She is now feeling healthy, looks great and claims to be living a higher quality life-style. I am very proud of her. She took control of her life and improved it greatly, and because of this new healthy life-style, she is actually increasing her longevity!

CHAPTER 32

Return to Youth Using Reflexology

The best road to perfect health and youthfulness is to give yourself a complete reflexology workout. Thoroughly work *all* the reflexes, to every gland and organ in your body. Special stimulation needs to be given to any reflex that is sore. Never overlook the importance of the endocrine glands. All these glands must be in perfect working order to keep you physically energized and mentally alert.

Remember that the adrenal glands control your energy and the drive to action. Your thyroid needs to be functioning well or your whole system will be sluggish. Keep from feeling tired and help all hormone-producing organs work well so that you will have renewed youthfulness and can live an active invigorating life. See Diagram 2.

REBUILD HEALTHY NEW CELLS

You can protect yourself from aging by using nature's wonderful healing forces to promote cellular regeneration. Each of the trillions of cells in your body is a living entity. You will age as slowly—or as rapidly—as each cell regenerates. When waste and toxins accumulate in the tissues, they interfere with the growth and development of the cells and the normal process of cell replacement. Adequate nourishment of the cells and sufficient oxygenation are not possible when waste and toxins are present. Cells that are not nourished sufficiently can cause premature aging and illness.

Use reflexology to rebuild healthy new cells by reactivating the organs of elimination, which are the lungs, liver, kidneys, and skin. Look at the zone therapy chart (Diagram 16) and work the reflexes to stimulate these organs. When you use reflex pressure in the corresponding zones, much of the accumulated waste and toxins will quickly be expelled from your body. As you restore a normal metabolic rate and cell oxygenation, new cells will replace the old ones. Renewed cells will produce renewed tissue, and this means a refreshingly younger and healthier new body.

STRENGTHEN YOUR DIGESTIVE SYSTEM

A sluggish metabolism and constipation will cause retention and accumulation of toxic wastes in the tissues which can cause many health problems and a feeling of weakness. Work the reflexes to the intestines, colon, and kidneys with a firm, rolling pressure, so that the natural circulation can be restored and lessen the obstruction to good health and youthfulness. See Diagrams 3 and 5.

Stimulate your digestive system with exercise. One that works well, is to place the Magic Reflex Massager in the palm of your left hand, place your right hand over it and squeeze your hands together as hard as you can. Feel your chest tighten up? Be consciously aware of your stomach muscles too, and tighten them during this exercise. This will strengthen a sluggish digestive system and firm up your tummy at the same time. This exercise works best when you are standing.

STAY YOUNG FOREVER

I am going to show you how you can electrify and revitalize your body and your life. No longer will you need to complain of fatigue which keeps you from doing the things you have always wanted to do. You will feel completely energized when you give your reflexes a brisk stimulating workout. One good exercise is a vigorous rub to all reflexes on the feet. See exercise and Photo "G." This exercise and the one to follow will stimulate the nerve impulses and renew every cell and organ with vibrant new energy.

After you have given your feet a vigorous rub hold your left foot under the heel with one hand, using the other hand to tap, or spank, the bottom, top and sides of your foot. Now using your thumb and index finger in a pinching position, press and slightly roll or twist each toe, from side to side—then work the tips of each toe. Exercise your foot at the ankle—push your toes forward and then backward, turn your foot to the left, then to the right—now make big circles to the left, then to the right. Finish this exercise by pounding your heels on the floor to stimulate circulation and renew energy throughout your body. See Photo 50. You will feel a tingling sensation as the circulation invigorates you to provide new cellular action. Soon you will look and feel the benefits of youthful vitality.

Dried Alfalfa Leaves Work Wonders

In the best of circumstances, we should all live to be about 120 years old. In Tibet there are people who are reportedly living to be 125 years old. They attribute their longevity to blood circulation and the daily consumption of herbs. The favorite herb of the Tibetan people is alfalfa. It is the only known plant that contains every nutrient that we need for growth and health. Alfalfa is a great remedy for high blood pressure, and it contains all the necessary elements needed for softening hard arteries. It is rich in iron, which helps with blood problems such as anemia; it contains potassium, for tissue and skin; and calcium, so you can be sure that it is an asset to bones and teeth.

Alfalfa works wonders with the liver and bowels to detoxify the body; is very effective for those who suffer from arthritis; is good for pituitary and hormone-producing glands; acts rapidly to alkalize the body; and is very beneficial in healing colds, bladder, and kidney problems. Alfalfa contains all the known vitamins, even the uncommon ones such as vitamins K, B-8, and U for peptic ulcers. I find it very interesting that it even contains phosphorus, which studies have shown will speed up the brain vibrations. It also supplies the blood with the necessary chemicals to produce keratin, one of the proteins found in hair. Reports from South Africa tell us that ostriches that were fed alfalfa produced stronger babies and their feathers had extremely brilliant and beautiful new color.

A treasure of nutritive elements is found in alfalfa. One of the reasons is that its roots go so deep and spread so wide that it absorbs a lot of valuable minerals and nourishment from the soil. Alfalfa can be purchased in tablet form. (If you are pregnant or nursing, consult your health care professional before using.) Alfalfa together with reflexology can increase your body's durability and at the same time invigorate your mind. This is a very exciting combination that will no doubt add health and youthfulness to your life.

These are not the same as alfalfa sprouts and remember, the best vitamins for "youthfulness" are vitamins C and E.

You can live to be a hundred years plus, too. All you have to do is consume a nutritious diet, exercise to maintain cardiovascular endurance, and use reflexology to heal ailing glands, organs, and muscles to promote renewed health, vigor, and youthfulness.

Reflexology Helps Rejuvenate Body and Mind

There is one very convenient point you can reach the moment you need additional mental energy. This special button is located beneath your nose, just above your upper lip. See Diagram 12 and Photo "H." When pressing this reflex you will be sending a force of life's energy to the pineal and pituitary glands (which are in the brain) and to the spleen and pancreas (to help blood and insulin levels). Work this "combination reflex" button with a gentle pressing, rolling motion as though you are rubbing the bone area under the skin. (Using knuckles is also effective on this reflex.) Press and rub for a slow count of seven, and then slowly release pressure for seven seconds. Repeat several times to strengthen and restore your mental energy.

At the same time, take a few slow deep breaths. The combination of new oxygen in your system and the stimulation of this special button will bring you renewed alertness and a quick mental lift. As you revive your mental awareness, your confidence will improve, and soon you will feel and look younger. Mental and physical health are both necessary to pursue your goals and attain the good life that you deserve.

Another method for quick mental alertness is to lie down on your bed, hang your head over the edge for five minutes, and take a few deep breaths. This will bring a new vigorous blood supply directly to your brain. Repeat four times a day when your intellect is challenged.

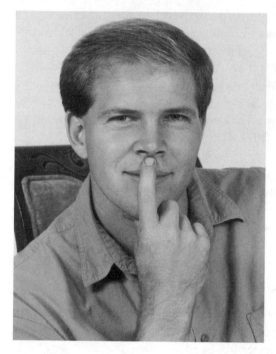

Photo "H": This reflex stimulates mental abilities. Helps improve alertness and memory. Also benefits some types of paralysis.

Breathe Your Way to Youthfulness

Reflexology and deep, natural breathing will do wonders for maintaining your youthfulness and good health. Use this combination to improve your immune power, balance your blood pressure, and keep your entire cardiovascular and respiratory systems working properly.

Unless provided with sufficient oxygen, your cells and every system in your body will become depleted, tired, and lifeless. As a result, you will lose your youthfulness and vitality. You need to take in at least seventy deep breaths every day, but work up to this. The effort is worth your time if you want to be young and healthy for the rest of your life.

Let me tell you about a very effective deep breathing exercise to use when you become tired. It is a bit unusual; however, it will quickly energize your body and stimulate your mind. I often use this secret method to boost my mental abilities.

Inhale a nice big breath through the nose; press your lips closely to the teeth, leaving open a very small space between your lips. Now exhale forcefully through this little space, using several very short bursts of air. Exhale all the air. (You will be able to hear these distinct bursts of air as they pass through your lips.) Relax and breathe normally for about thirty seconds, then repeat. However, do *not* overdue this exercise at first, and if by chance you feel faint or dizzy, sit down and do not continue. Return to your relaxed deep breathing.

Deep breathing with your reflex workout will be soothing, relaxing, and very enjoyable. It will leave you feeling extremely rested and never tense or sore. Take an active role in your own health and pride in your body by using reflexology to control any possible decline in age.

DRINK WATER TO STAY YOUNG AND HEALTHY

Did you know that drinking a glass of pure water will energize your whole system? Water is nature's very own youth builder, and it will keep you from aging. It helps your body function in almost every way. It improves digestive efficiency, helps kidneys flush out toxins, prevents constipation, and rebuilds your immune system. Water hydrates your skin and hair to keep you looking young and healthy. You will want to drink six to eight glasses everyday, more if you are overweight.

You will be surprised at how fast your energy returns and your performance improves when your body receives sufficient amounts of fresh, clean, rejuvenating water.

REFLEXOLOGY FOR BETTER SPORTS PERFORMANCE

Reflexology used along with endurance-building exercises will improve the functions of the heart, lungs, and blood vessels. Keep your blood vessels free of obstructions through reflex massage, and you will experience renewed strength. Fresh blood nourishes billions of body cells and gives your whole system an invigorating blast of health and energy.

Work the reflexes to your lungs and vascular network to keep your circulatory system working at its peak. In addition to your daily reflex workout, remember to keep your joints flexible and muscles elastic by stretching, bending, walking, and moving about. Athletes, dancers, and those involved in programs of physical fitness will all benefit from regular reflex workouts.

Reflexology Benefits Body Builder and Runner

Dear Mrs. Carter,

I enjoy massaging my sciatic nerve reflex. In the past, when I worked my legs in body building, they would get sore the next day. Since I have been massaging my legs, ankles, and heels on both legs, I never get sore any more. Even my knees are no longer sore when I do deep knee bends. Mrs. Carter, I would have to write a book to explain what reflexology did for me. Thank you for writing such wonderful books.

—T.C.

Reflexologists are often found at marathons and other sporting events, helping when needed. A man who knew nothing of reflexology was running in a marathon and his back started hurting him. He told me later that "someone" asked if they could help him. He agreed, and before he knew what was happening, he was getting a reflexology treatment on his hand. He said that the reflexologist worked the back of his hand, down his index finger to the wrist for a few minutes, then showed him how to work this reflex on himself if he needed it later in the run. He took off running again, felt great, and didn't think about his back again until after the marathon. "I will never forget what a difference that volunteer reflexologist made in my day!" he told me.

MAKE THE CHOICE TO STAY YOUNG AND WELL

Work the reflex to your lymph glands and spleen to keep your immune system active and strong. See Diagrams 3, 4, 5, and 12. The more powerful your immune system is, the less chance infectious organisms have of surviving. The cells that attack and wipe out invaders are the same cells that protect you against aging. Your body needs active lymphocytes to keep you young and well.

Make the choice to stay healthy, young, and pain free by using the magic massager with the little fingers. It will stimulate the reflexes in your hands and send a flow of energized electrical life forces throughout most of the organs and glands in your whole body. You can take it with you wherever you go; keep one with you at work or put one in your pocket and use it when standing in a shopping line. At home you can place it under your foot, rolling it underneath. Soon you will feel refreshed and rejuvenated. See Photo 48.

How Laughing and Smiling Keep You Young

Laughter will energize your whole system as it accelerates your heart rate and respiration. A good laugh will release adrenaline for fast energy and will stimulate and motivate a person who feels depressed. It brings fresh air into the lungs which also increases your level of energy. Laughter is very healing to your whole body and will renew each cell and organ with vibrancy. See Photo "I".

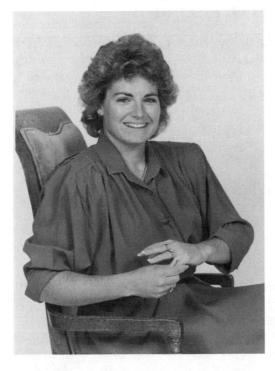

Photo "I": Stay young with laughter, and renew your energy by applying pressure to the little finger.

In addition to the "do-it-yourself face lift" exercises (Chapter 34), smiling will keep your face radiant and youthful.

Your face has several muscles that help express emotion. When you are happy and smile, the facial and neck muscles are uplifted. When you laugh very hard, you can feel the muscles working as they tighten and relax. Take a moment and smile; notice how the muscles from your scalp pull up on the muscles in your forehead. The muscles in your cheeks pull your lips up and out, and the muscles attached to your chest tighten the neck. When you laugh hard, the jaw muscles are exercised as you open your mouth, and you can feel your upper lip move upward. Even the muscles around the eyes get a workout.

Keep in mind that a sad or angry expression will pull the muscles down, creating frown lines. As one gets older, their habitual expressions will be visible on their face, revealing which muscles were used the most. So make the choice to smile and laugh. Like reflexology, this method of revitalizing your life can be used anytime, and anyplace, and costs you nothing.

A Sampling of Letters From and About Readers Over Eighty

I would like to share with you a few letters that I have received from readers who are over eighty years old.

Reflexology Helped Pain Vanish and I Slept Soundly

Dear Mrs. Carter,

While my street was being widened and paved, I was climbing over the ditches in the dark, and I pulled a muscle or tendon on the inside of the right femur. I played bridge that night, and it hurt every time I got up to move. The next day the pain continued and by 6 P.M., I simply could not walk without holding onto chairs. I was positively ill with pain. I went to bed with the electric pad under me, but that did no good. Finally *reflexology* came to mind. I decided to simply hunt for a tender spot on my right foot and found one at once, and worked on it for a very few minutes. I went off to sleep and slept soundly all night. (Usually get up once or twice each night.) In the morning the pain was *gone*. I am 84 years of age.

Sincerely,

—B.B.

Mother-in-Law Saved from Nursing Home

Dear Mildred Carter,

Enclosed find a picture of my mother-in-law who came to live with us over five years ago. She had complete heart failure, three strokes, high blood pressure, diabetes, and cancer in her breast. Our doctor told us to put her in a nursing home as her life span was about over, but we kept her, and I used reflexology on her. I have had the book for years. Mom has not had a cold in five years, eats, sleeps, and enjoys life and never sees a bad day. I take her twice a year for a physical, and the doctors say "I don't know what you are doing, but keep up the good work." They can't find any heart trouble, her lungs are good, and the cancer has not moved or given her any trouble.

This is a true story, and mom will be eighty-three years old this December.

—A student

How Reflexology Helped a Ninety-five-Year-Old with World War I Disabilities

Dear Mrs. Carter,

I am ninety-five years old and almost bedridden with permanent World War I disabilities. Within the last two years I suffered a fall and head injury, had brain surgery, then a heart attack, a stroke, and later another stroke. Then I had food poisoning and had to have my stomach pumped. Struggling alone while having to use a walker has been a challenge, but I feel with the help of reflexology and good nutrition, I can go on for another sixty years. I believe anyone can have success with reflexology.

Reflex massage has helped me with so many of my physical problems. I have used it for foot pain, heart pains, anxiety, reduced circulation and numbness in my legs and arms, and boosting my entire immune system.

Divine love to you and yours. You are fantastically gifted in healing.

—Mr. S.H.

CHAPTER 33

How Reflexology Helps the Athlete

Reflexology is nature's "push button" secret for dynamic living, abundant physical energy, vibrant health, youthful vigor, and the *sole* way to a better athlete! Yes . . . reflexology on the sole of your feet will help you stay in good shape, naturally. Peak performance is what every athlete strives to attain. And in order to achieve your maximum goal, you must be completely healthy . . . physically, mentally and emotionally.

Reflexology is a scientific technique that has a definite effect on the functioning of all glands and organs. It sends a healing energy through the body, which travels on specific zone pathways, called "life force" or "vital energy" channels. See Diagram 16.

WHAT EVERY ATHLETE MUST KNOW

Every sports enthusiast, from the weekend athletes right on up to the pros . . . depend on good physical abilities and sharp mental skills to help them play well and win. Whether you are skiing down a powdery slope . . . ready to hit the ball . . . or make a putt, you must be in top form for every move. Reflexology is a great benefit to any sport and can be used by people of all ages. A complete reflex workout will tune up your body and give you that extra go power and vitality needed for winning. Also it will improve your mental allertness, which helps prevent accidents, and give you more confidence.

Make reflexology part of your weekly regimen. Study this book and heed the cautions. You will not want to overdo it the first few times.

Whether you play baseball, contact sports, racquet sports, field sports, ski or swim . . . you depend on good vision and hearing, to be at your competitive best. Work the reflexes to eyes and ears to ensure good sight and sound. See Diagram 3 and 5.

Fifteen Ways the Athlete Can Benefit from Reflexology

1. Promotes good circulation
2. Stimulates stamina
3. Balances vital energies
4. Increases endurance
5. Revitalizes the power of concentration
6. Helps cleanse body of toxins and impurities
7. Helps the body heal more quickly
8. Opens and clears neural pathways
9. Renews physical health
10. Helps the body restore youthful vitality
11. Activates the nervous system
12. Reduces stress and tension
13. Improves mental energy
14. Induces tranquil relaxation
15. Reflexology feels wonderful, and costs nothing!

YOUR BODY AND ITS "TEAM" OF INTER-RELATED SYSTEMS

First, let us give our attention to the all-important endocrine glands. These glands are all interrelated and supplement and depend on each other. Their normal functions and development are of great importance to the well-being of every sports enthusiast. All athletes need to keep these glands tuned up, for they influence, not only your health, but your body growth, muscle/nerve operation, heartbeat, control blood sugar, promote courage and produce adrenalin for extra energy and drive. These are just a few of the important reasons you must keep this system working harmoniously. See Diagram 2.

Of course, all systems are interrelated. Single cells do not function by themselves, nor do body systems operate independently. Reflexology will activate healing powers to every area of the body, and balance the whole system. Although there are thousands of parts, each with its own purpose, they all work together to make one complete body. (What a great team!) This is why a COMPLETE workout on all reflexes is very important. Keep your body healthy and balanced so it will be ready for the ultimate challenge. See Diagrams 3 and 5.

INCREASE YOUR ENERGY FOR PEAK PERFORMANCE

The most imporant thing to a good athlete is endurance and stamina. Being able to keep up with everyone else is of utmost importance. Reflexology stimulates the vital life force for renewed energy. Your body is designed to construct, and reconstruct itself. It is forever changing, and you play the major role in maintaining it.

A nutricious diet and exercise is of utmost importance to keep bones and muscles strong and healthy. Reflexology gets the circulation moving, so that blood delivers sufficient minerals and oxygen to the cells of the muscles and bones. Without vital nutrients neither the muscles, nor the bones will be strong enough for vigorous activity.

When You Need Additional Energy

A reflex workout is a great way to gain that additional blast of energy, known as the *second wind*. You will feel properly charged as you bring forth that reserve of vim and vigour.

One pressure point to work when you need additional pep in your step, is the pituitary reflex. This reflex is located on each of your thumbs. Also, press and pinch your little fingers, then give your entire hand, both front and back, a vigorous rub to stimulate energy. Clapping hands together also generates energy. If you enjoy a barefoot sport, such as jogging on the beach, swimming or surfing, you can reach down and give each of your feet a vigorous rub. Give your pituitary button on each big toe a little extra attention, too.

Another fast workout for extra energy, is to take your thumb, or use a strong knuckle, and press into the center of your palm on the opposite hand. Use a rolling, pressing motion, you will be sending vital energy to the adrenal reflex . . . beneficial for a renewed boost of adrenalin. The magic massager will cover these reflexes quite satisfactorily, if you have one. Remember not to overstimulate this area the first few times, as working this area also stimulates the more sensitive organs and glands in your body.

BREATHE COLOR TO INCREASE ENERGY

If you really want to be a human dynamo, then follow this method. Evelyn Monahan gives us a great technique for using color to build unending energy.

First, you lie down or sit in a straight back chair with a head rest so that you can completely relax. Now, with the power of your mind, picture the color of a bright beautiful *red*. Close your eyes and picture this red surrounding you. When you are enveloped in the color red and you are completely relaxed, start breathing this color into your lungs, using the yoga breathing that I described earlier. When your lungs are full of this red, relax your stomach muscles, still holding the red breath. Now, picture the red flowing through your whole body, send it down to the ends of your toes and then bring it back up and run it slowly through every part of your body, including your head.

Now you should feel as if your whole body is enveloped in the color red. When you release the red air, you will release it out through every part of your body. Do this three times. Then, while still relaxed, you will repeat to yourself mentally: "Through the use of my energized mind, I am able to take full advantage of the limitless energy which the universal blueprint of redness makes available to me. My mind and body are flooded with infinite energy and all tiredness and fatigue have left me and been replaced with an inexhaustible supply of pure energy. My high self will keep me in constant touch with my own source of infinite power."

Again, you will take in the deep breath filled with red, relaxing the stomach muscles and then following the red throughout the body as you did the first time—releasing the air through the whole of your body but retaining the color red. Repeat this three times.

As you feel the flow of the color red traveling through your body, picture and feel the energy you are receiving from it. With practice, you will soon become very adept with this technique of building an inexhaustible supply of energy and you need never be tired again. It works! I use this color technique often to help keep me on top of my heavy work schedule.

Like reflexology, this method of revitalizing your energy can be used anytime and anywhere and costs you nothing.

HELP FOR BRUISES AND INJURIES

When using reflexology, tiny invisible electrical impulses are sent through to the corresponding gland or organ, thus nature has the opportunity to restore and renew your body, both mentally and physically.

Reflex pressure is NEVER to be used on cuts, blisters, scrapes or broken bones. See a licensed doctor for serious injuries. If one does become laid up for a few days, it could be beneficial to stimulate the lymph nodes, which keep the immune system healthy and heal infections in the body. Together the liver, spleen and lymph system filter out bacteria.

One easy exercise is to elevate feet, and "pump your lymph nodes" . . . point your toes forward and then backward, then from side to side, roll ankles in circles to the left, then right. Do the same exercise with hands to help nature eliminate congestion and infection from all parts of the body.

Use RICE for Sprains, Strains, and Tendinitis

There is a common procedure called RICE, which is often used if someone gets a sprain or strain during a sports event. You can easily remember it by learning: R . . means *Rest* the injured area; I . . means to apply *Ice* to the part that is injured for 10 to 20 minutes, remove and re-apply every two waking hours for the next two days. C . . is for *Compression,* which can be used, (however, not too tightly or circulation will be cut off) a towel or soft cloth works well when placed around the injury. E . . is to *Elevate* the injured part above the heart.

How to Stop a Calf Cramp Immediately

The dorsiflex, (bringing toes toward nose) has helped stop many calf cramps during sports events, or at nightime. It is also very helpful if you happen to have sciatic nerve pain in your lower leg. Fast action will reduce nerve tension and help the leg to relax.

You can stop a cramp or "charlie-horse" within five seconds, providing you take action immediately. At the first twinge of tightness in your calf, stretch your leg out straight, then , at the same time, bend your foot at the ankle, push your heel away from your body and point your toes toward your nose (this will extend your calf muscles). Hold this position until all pain is gone. It may feel good to also gently massage the calf muscles.

Badminton Champion Back on His Feet

Dear Mrs. Carter,

I have used reflexology on myself and others with great success. I have worked on some spectacular cases that were against all medical odds! What reflexology does is positively startling . . . even the impossible becomes possible. Take for instance the singles badminton champion, Mr. P.S., who was half-paralyzed from the shoulder to the toe and had been bed-ridden for six long years. With the use of reflexology, this man fought against medical odds to bring circulation back in his life again. In less than four months, his paralyzed conditions had improved tremendously. Mr. P.S. was a perfectionist and with the special effects of reflexology he can now walk without the aid of a walking stick.

Sportsmen must be fit, but they cannot be if their biological functions are improper. Reflexology insures that the body is a well oiled and smooth running "machine".

—B.C.

Coach Uses Reflexology

Dear Ms. Carter,

Since I have been a physcial education teacher and coach for 31 years, I am well aware of having a positive outlook toward life and maintaining a good self-image in handling whatever life seems to put into our paths. I do believe in a power greater than myself and I always try to maintain and pass onto others the idea that no matter what happens to us there is a reason and we must try to rise above it and grow as a result of the situation. I have used reflexology to help those who suffer pain and have seen very good results.

—M.K.

CHAPTER 34

Reflexology's Sensational Way to Beauty

We all want to be beautiful from the time we are small children until we become centenarians. *You are beautiful!* Maybe you don't think you are, but you are truly beautiful, and I am going to show you how to bring your true beauty out into the open where it shows.

Perfect health is the first requirement for beauty. To be beautiful, you must radiate health. I will give you a new way to capture vibrant health and beauty you never dreamed was possible, if you will only follow my directions. To be radiantly beautiful, you will have to be radiantly healthy and beautiful on the inside. You already know how to use reflexology massage to turn a tired, sick body into one vibrant with energy and health. Now, let us turn to reflex therapy to give you a perfect petal-smooth skin and to keep it beautiful for the rest of your life.

Of first importance is to have the endocrine glands in good condition. Keep them healthy by massaging the reflexes to these glands. See Diagram 2.

AID TO SKIN BEAUTY

Because I have always had very sensitive skin and all soaps and cosmetics caused a rash, I searched for many years to find the perfect lotion to bring out the beauty of my skin and keep it beautiful. In my search for a healing, moisturizing skin lotion that contained only pure natural ingredients, I discovered *aloe vera*, the miracle plant. Ancient aloe vera juice has incredible benefits. I combined it with modern vitamin E and other rich emollients to banish such common skin problems as wrinkles, blemishes, age lines, dry flaky skin, brown spots, crepey throat, and acne and to help the skin retain moisture.

Aloe vera is a genus of plant belonging to the lily family. It is a succulent plant, originally from North Africa, used throughout the world as nature's miracle healing plant. For more than three thousand years, aloe vera reportedly has been used for medicinal purposes. One of the earliest written references to this plant is in the Bible, John 19:39. In biblical times aloes were very valuable. It is said that the women of ancient Egypt and Greece used the gel from the aloe vera plant to improve their complexions and skin textures. It is believed that Cleopatra's beauty can be credited to this plant.

Mildred Carter's Aloe Vera-E Cosmetics are available to you through Stirling Enterprises, Inc., Box 216, Cottage Grove, Oregon 97424.

A DO-IT-YOURSELF FACE LIFT AT HOME

Everyone hates to look in the mirror and see the lines of age start creeping into his or her face. More and more people are turning to cosmetic surgery to have these lines removed—if they can afford the price. Millions of dollars are spent on advertised skin remedies for trying to cover up these telltale signs of age. In previous chapters, I have told you how to work on certain reflexes to overcome every type of ailment. Now, I am going to tell you how you can use reflexology to give yourself an *at-home* face lift and keep that youthful look for the rest of your life. If you take the time and follow directions closely, you will be able to erase a decade of wrinkles, creases, and crow's feet. This treatment works especially well for middle-aged women and men. The earlier you work on your wrinkles, the greater your success.

With reflexology, you have a safe, simple, effective means of achieving a face lift without the risks of surgery—no painful postoperative period and no doctor's fees. You simply press certain reflex buttons on your face with your fingers and, over time, watch your wrinkles disappear!

Look at Photo 61 and notice how various points covering the face are numbered. When you use this pressure point technique, excessive muscle tone is relaxed and sagging muscle tone is tightened. You will have to follow the pressing and tapping of these certain buttons on your face for a specified time. For the first five weeks, do this special reflex method three times a week. For the next three weeks, do the exercise two times a week. Then, once a week for the next two weeks. After this, put yourself on a maintenance schedule of once every two weeks.

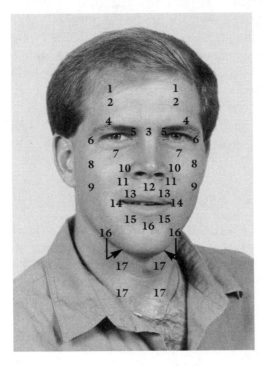

Photo 61: The numbers on the face indicate how you can give yourself a reflexology "face lift" at home by pressing and tapping certain reflex buttons.

Many experts agree that you can reduce wrinkles and improve your looks with this technique of face reflexology. They also agree that dry skin is a major cause of the skin wrinkling. While using this method of face reflexology, it is of the greatest importance to use moisturizing creams to achieve the best results. This is where my Aloe Vera-E lotions will help keep your skin soft and moist twenty-four hours a day.

This unique system is so effective because we relax and remove tension, then create sound waves from tapping with the fingers to help improve circulation and give a nutritive oxygen supply to skin and cells, which is invaluable for a smoother and more radiant looking skin. Small sound waves actually help the skin cells to exercise, which will tone and restore the muscles to prevent lines and wrinkles. Underlying muscles that may have lost their elasticity will soon restore supportive structure and become more youthful looking.

Relaxing and Toning the Reflex Buttons

Sit in a comfortable chair. Have a watch with a second hand ready to time yourself. Notice in Photo 61 that the reflex buttons are clearly numbered for each wrinkle group. Most buttons will be on both sides of your face, so use both hands simultaneously.

This method of rebuilding sagging face muscles is different from massaging the reflexes in the face for stimulating certain glands and organs in the body. This natural face-lift treatment will involve relaxing and toning each of the buttons listed.

First, we will *relax and remove tension*. Using the pads of the middle fingers, press firmly and deeply enough to create mild discomfort, hold for ten seconds, then gradually release the pressure for ten seconds. Repeat this procedure six times; this will total two minutes.

Next *tighten the skin* by toning the button. Tap the area lightly with the fingertips for ten seconds, then pause ten seconds. Repeat this procedure three times. This will total one minute.

After every set of exercises, move your hands away from your body and shake them loosely to release tension.

If you do all the exercises, it will take approximately an hour. Can you afford an hour three times a week to regain a beautiful, firm, youthful complexion?

You do not have to do the whole face lift procedure. Maybe you have only one or two sets of wrinkles to overcome, such as on the forehead or around the eyes. This procedure would only take a few minutes.

Stay comfortable and relaxed, and breathe deeply. Also remember to drink plenty of water to keep your skin hydrated; this will help keep it moist and resilient. We will work on seventeen buttons to eliminate wrinkles on the entire face and neck.

Let us start with the wrinkles on the forehead, pressure point 1, then follow the rest of the chart below.

Tehnique:

> *Step 1:* Press firmly and hold for 10 seconds; pause for 10 seconds. Repeat 6 times.

> *Step 2:* Tap lightly for 10 seconds; pause for 10 seconds. Repeat 3 times.

> *Step 3:* Shake hands loosely for 5 seconds, then proceed to next button.

"DO IT YOURSELF" FACE LIFT LOCATION CHART

Location	Theory	Pressure Points
Wrinkles on forehead	Helps firm furrowed brow	1, 2
Wrinkles on bridge of nose	Erases lines across bridge of nose	3
Wrinkles around eyes	Vanishes upper and lower eye wrinkles and crow's feet	4, 5, 6, 7
Face wrinkles (including laugh lines)	Tones and tightens cheek and jaw area while pressing out laugh lines	8, 9, 10, 11
Wrinkles around mouth	Dissolves laugh lines and adds firmness to lips	12, 13, 14, 15
Chin and under chin	Tones chin for a youthful appearance. Stimulates glands for a beautiful complexion.	*16
Neck	Renews muscle tone to control double chin	17

* An additional firming exercise for the chin and neck is to gently tap with the back of your hands rhythmically beneath the chin in an outward rotating motion (30 seconds).

Addition to "Do It Yourself" Face Lift

Now, you have covered all the face muscles to give you an easy and simple at-home face lift, and no one need be the wiser. It will take some of your time, but think how rewarding it will be when your friends start asking you what you have done to look so young! When you use my special exotic aloe vera moisturizing lotions along with the special face lift, you will have a million-dollar secret to keep you young-looking and beautiful the rest of your life.

Protect Your Skin from Wrinkles

To protect your skin and keep your face free from wrinkles, sleep on a satin pillowcase. Your face will glide over the satin, instead of being pulled out of shape by the rough texture of a cotton pillowcase. Make sure your pillow is not too firm, or your head will slide off the smooth satin.

Pulling Ears for Beauty

I have explained in Chapter 4 on ears how beneficial it is to pull on the ears to help stimulate many organs and glands, especially those that influence the skin. See Photos 18, 19, and 20.

Reflexes to Hormone-Producing Glands

Place your thumbs just under both sides of the chin. See Photo 25. With your thumbs hooked under your chin, work on your lymph nodes to make this area soft and pliable. This will increase both energy and the flow of hormones. The skin will be able to breathe so you will have healthier skin with wrinkles gone and less need for cosmetics. Your skin will also be easier to shave. Press in with the thumbs, and milk these glands toward the chin. Do this one at a time about three times on each side.

The next method of reflex massage helps even quite elderly women and men remain wrinkle-free and beautiful. Place the thumb on one side of the esophagus (throat) and the fingers on the opposite side. See Photo 30. Starting under the chin, press and massage with a rolling motion all the way to the collarbone. Then change hands and do it with the opposite thumb and fingers. Do this three times with each hand. Now use the same procedure, only start at the collarbone and massage up toward the chin three times with each hand. This also will stimulate the production of hormones, giving you a beautiful complexion.

A Touch for Beauty

See the numbered reflex buttons on the face in Photo 62. With the ring finger, start on number 1 at the top of the forehead. With a gentle, rolling pressure, massage this reflex for the count of three; then repeat the procedure with numbers 2 and 3. For numbers 4, 5, and 6, use the fingers of both hands simultaneously. Continue with one finger on 7, 8, and 9. Do this twice a day when you are cleaning your face, and let it become a habit, to stimulate beauty and health-producing hormones throughout the body.

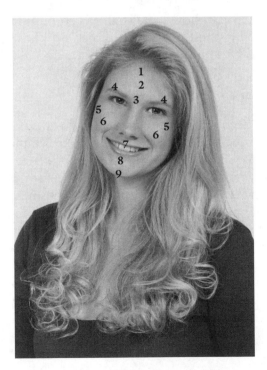

Photo 62: The numbers on the face indicate special reflex buttons that will aid in developing a beautiful complexion.

I have given you several ways to help regain beautiful skin and to keep it healthy and beautiful the rest of your life by using the touch of your fingertips. Always remember your true beauty comes from within, no matter what methods you use to beautify your body on the outside. If your heart is filled with envy, hate, jealousy, and ugly, unhappy thoughts, it will discolor your aura for all to see.

What you thought yesterday, you will live today, what you think today, you will live tomorrow. If you want to live a life filled with health and beauty, joy, and happiness, then think *only* of that which is beautiful! And you *will* be *beautiful.*

HELP FOR ACNE

The heartbreak of many a young developing boy and girl is acne, the problems of which sometimes, psychologically, last into adult life. Acne is not cured from the outside alone. You must treat the cause, and diet is at the root of the cause. You need to eat lots of raw vegetables and fruits instead of starches and sugars. Take lots of vitamins A, C, and B vitamins. Get lots of good hard exercise to get oxygen into the bloodstream.

The trampoline is especially good to get oxygen circulating through every cell in your body. The miniature trampoline called the rebounder is described in this book in Chapter 36, on using reflex devices.

Use reflexology on all the reflexes to the endocrine glands, to stimulate oil and hormones into the skin. See Diagram 2. Remember, a healthy body means a healthy skin and a beautiful complexion.

I am going to give you a sure cure for acne, for getting at the cause on the inside. This is a recipe using brewer's yeast, which abounds in B vitamins. Start with a small amount and increase it up to the amount in the recipe.

> Take one to two tablespoons of brewer's yeast, which can be found at the health food store (not baker's yeast), one to two tablespoons lecithin or two lecithin capsules (I like to use the capsules), one tablespoon cold pressed oil (safflower oil preferred). Take with milk, nonfat dairy milk, or apple juice. If you wish to add a sweetener, do not use sugar but a substitute. I like to use blackstrap molasses,

which not only sweetens but also is filled with minerals and is healthy for you. Take this every morning and add vitamins and calcium.

If you stay with this recipe and don't neglect taking it every day, this will not only turn you into a human dynamo of energy and happiness, it will also reward you with a beautiful, clear complexion and glossy healthy hair. If you go on a trip, a long one or just overnight, take your brewer's yeast with you.

I would advise you to use only pure soaps. (I never use soap on my face.) You might want to use my special skin lotions which are developed from aloe vera and vitamin E to help develop and keep a silky smooth complexion the rest of your life.

How to Remove Acne Scars

Aloe vera is very effective in gradually reducing old acne scars if used over a period of time. You may want to get a plant of your own and harvest the leaves. Cut the leaves closest to the ground, as these are the oldest and most potent medicinally. You need only a little gel from the cut end of the leaf. (Wrap the rest of the leaf in a zip lock baggie and put it into the refrigerator for later use.) Apply a thin layer over the skin twice a day for as long as it takes. In addition, use a natural fruit peel to continuously exfoliate and encourage new skin. If scars are deep, it may take a year to grow all the new skin needed, but this is a project that will be well worth the wait. Aloe vera acts as an astringent to reduce oily skin. So if you have dry skin, you will want to use my special exotic moisturizing creams along with the aloe vera gel. ALWAYS protect new skin from harmful rays of the sun with a natural mineral sunscreen.

HOW TO CONTROL PSORIASIS AND ECZEMA

Psoriasis is not contagious and it can be controlled. It is a persistent skin condition that needs both internal and external attention. Often emotional or physical stress cause greater problems, and some people claim their ailment worsens during the winter months.

Normal skin cells will live for about one month, then dry up and flake off. The skin cells with psoriasis seem to dry up and flake off in about five days, leaving thick, red eruptions, sometimes covered by silvery scales. Psoriasis usually appears on the bottom of the feet, palm of the hands, back, buttocks, elbows, knees, or scalp. If it spreads to the fingernails, they may fray or thicken and often will become discolored.

Carla's Summer Vacation

Last summer I treated a teenage girl who was the niece of a neighbor. Carla was visiting for a week and had planned to ride horses, swim, and hike with the girls she had met on her vacation here last year. But instead of having fun with her friends, she was indoors and quite miserable from an intolerable skin rash. This adorable little girl was itching constantly at the rough, cracked, and bleeding eruptions on her hands and elbows.

Reflexology is not an overnight cure for psoriasis, but I knew it would help balance her system and relax her. So I worked the reflexes on her feet, and at the same time, taught her to breathe deeply. I explained to her how deep breathing affects the richness of blood, which is the basis of the skin's natural health.

Carla seemed to sleep a lot, which is very beneficial when the body is healing itself, and new cells are being made to replace the old used cells. So we let her sleep all she wanted. We cleansed her skin around the affected area to prevent infection, then applied vitamin E oil. Her skin was sensitive, so we did not rub it in. We simply coated the area very lightly with a thin layer.

To increase the natural flow of energy throughout her body, we gave her a complete reflex workout on her feet. For dinner Carla had cottage cheese with a half teaspoon of flax oil and a half teaspoon cod-liver oil (the cottage cheese helps the oil bind better, and the body will absorb it much more readily). Both oils are good for skin disorders. Flax oil is especially helpful to stop the itching. Carla also had a fruit drink with one tablespoon of lecithin mixed in, which is beneficial to healing disorders of the skin—and a vitamin E tablet which should always be taken with lecithin. Read why on page 119.

The next morning Carla reported that she did not feel the need to itch so often. Her aunt gave her a bowl of oatmeal with the oil mixture added and some lecithin granules sprinkled on top, with a glass of juice and a vitamin E tablet. She worked Carla's foot reflexes for thirty minutes.

For the next two days, my neighbor continued to apply vitamin E every four hours and worked Carla's feet for thirty minutes every morning, reminding her to breathe deeply. She gave her nutritious meals and encouraged the afternoon naps.

After three days of treatment, adding vitamin E to her skin, oils and lecithin to her diet, and lots of rest, Carla was riding horses and hiking with her friends. The skin disorder was not completely gone; however, there were no new outbreaks and the itching had subsided. Carla was happily having the time of her life.

How Reflexology and Fish Oils Help the Skin

Reflexology will balance the body's chemistry when used to help psoriasis and eczematous rashes. A complete workout on both feet or both hands produces remarkable improvements.

It is important to concentrate on all the endocrine reflexes, as they are responsible for determining the forms of our bodies.

Work the liver reflex for seven to ten seconds on each hand or foot, as it helps supply substances for making good strong healing blood and is a great filter and a natural antiseptic. See Diagrams 3 and 5.

Also work the reflex to the kidneys, so they will filter and clean the blood. Your kidneys also keep proper water and acid balance in the body. (Studies show that foods containing pineapple, tomatoes, and other foods high in acids aggravate most skin disorders.) However, there are certain foods and food supplements that will help alleviate skin disorders. Foods such as sardines and salmon are rich in important nutrients, also supplements with natural fatty acids and fish oils are extremely beneficial. You might choose to take omega 3 oil, cod-liver oil, or Heralifeline with selected herbs. These are supplements which contain natural liquid marine lipids that provide a full spectrum of fatty acids.

Reflexology and fish oils are very beneficial for the heart. And a healthy heart is advantageous to healthy skin. Work the reflex to the heart and spleen. You will find these reflexes on the left foot and the left hand, at the outer edge (see Diagrams 3 and 5), and below your nose (see Photos "H" and 46). This will help maintain the process of producing antibodies and filtering the blood, as well as clearing out old blood cells, bacteria, and waste. Also spend a few extra minutes working the lymph glands. Look at Diagram 4 to see how the reflex to these little lymph nodes are all the way across the top of the foot and wrist. You are now strengthening nature in her efforts to heal the body's blood, nerves and tissues, thus bringing the whole body into perfect balance and health.

CHAPTER 35

How Reflexology Can Help Children

Children are the easiest subjects on whom to use reflexology since they are still attuned to nature and their natural instincts tell them this is the correct way to find healing for any ailments that they might have.

I have treated many children for various complaints with reflex therapy, and they have always benefited by the treatment. When I push a button that is really an ouch spot, the children will flinch a little but insist that I keep working. They know this is nature's way of overcoming any congestion that might be present in their bodies.

All children should be taught reflexology, not only to use on themselves, but also on others. You never know when their knowledge might save a life in future years; the life that is saved might be yours!

Children can learn to use the natural healing forces of reflexology to relieve pain from many sources in minutes, such as headache, toothache, nervous tension, and even the more serious illnesses such as a heart attack or a stroke, or traumas caused by an accident.

Any of the methods shown in this book may be used on children with a very gentle pressure, even on the body reflexes as shown in the charts. The only exception is the soft spot on top of a newborn's skull. NEVER use pressure here; this is where the four pieces of the bone have not yet grown together. It is protected by a tough membrane, which closes when the baby is between ten and twenty months old. Hand and foot reflexology may be used on very tiny babies. Use the amount of pressure you would use on the petal of a flower when you begin the reflex work, lightly increasing the pressure when you find a tender reflex. When you touch a tender reflex, the baby will flinch.

REFLEXOLOGY COMFORTS BABIES

I have seen many babies stop crying in minutes after reflexology was applied. One time my friend and I were traveling in the car and we stopped at a hotel restaurant for dinner. We had just been seated when two women came in with a little crying baby who was making a loud piercing sound. He was screaming at the top of his lungs. It looked like a mother and her daughter with a new baby. They kept handing him back and forth, trying to comfort him; however, he kept crying.

They sat at the table behind ours, and my friend went over to them and told them I was a reflexologist. We asked if they would like my help, and when they said they would, I took the baby's little bare foot in my hand and gently worked the bottom. He soon stopped crying and went to sleep. He was as tired as they were. All the people in the restaurant came rushing over. I think they thought we had killed him. As soon as I quit working his foot he woke up and starting screaming again. I showed the mother and grandmother how to rub his tiny little foot. They got him to sleep, ordered their dinner to be sent up to their room, and left with the sleeping baby. They said they were going to buy every book they could find on reflexology the very next day.

A very soft and lightly scratching movement on the back of the hands with the fingernails is very soothing and usually quiets a restless child. Research shows that in hospitals where premature babies are regularly touched, they progress much faster than do babies in hospitals where not much physical contact is allowed. One of my clients, Caroline, said that she'd had a colicky baby. It made her feel totally helpless and frustrated. After using the simple technique of reflexology, both she and the baby were able to sleep.

Caroline works part time at a medical clinic, and is very concerned with problems of the children who come in, especially those children who have been mistreated physically. She has a real passion for children and a great interest in reflexology. She strongly testifies that reflex therapy works wonders. With the loving contact of reflexology, both parent and child feel a closer bond, and both are able to relax more easily and feel a greater sense of security.

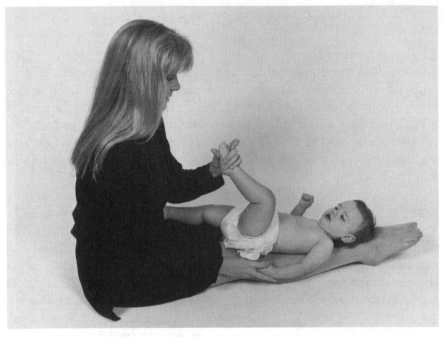

Photo "J": Lay baby on his/her back so you can see each other's facial expressions. Light pressure on baby's foot will bring harmony and good health.

HOW TO RELIEVE DIGESTIVE PROBLEMS

With your left hand open, gently press on the tummy. This reflex point is usually found about two inches below the navel. However, ask where it hurts and place the palm of your hand directly over this area. You may feel the pulse of blood at this point. Hold your hand there until the heat and warmth from it gives a sedating, soothing effect. There may be a sensation of cleansing as the digestive problems dissolve. See Photo 2.

The most effective use of reflexology is when one gives a complete reflex workout to all glands and organs to improve circulation and stimulate energy. However, if a child becomes ill, the first thing to turn to is the endocrine glands. Start on the reflexes in the big toes, or the thumbs. See the charts on the endocrine glands and learn the location of the reflexes to all these important hormone-producing organs. Remember, if just one of the endocrine glands is not functioning perfectly, it will throw all the other endocrine glands out of balance, thus causing disharmony in the whole body. See Diagram 2.

Many are concerned regarding the health and welfare of children. I receive many thankful letters from parents and friends of children. I would like to share a few with you.

Dear Mrs. Carter,

I like the way reflexology can be helpful without being expensive or harmful and can be used for family members and children. As a parent I like to help heal something before it gets serious and requires medical attention. I see this work becoming more popular all the time. It is knowledge in our minds that cannot be taken away by anyone else. It can be used almost anytime, almost anywhere.

—Mr. D.R.

Dear Mrs. Carter,

I have had so many wonderful experiences with reflexology—I now want to tell you about one girl, thirteen years old, that the doctors gave two weeks to live because she had tonsillitis poisoning and the doctors could not relieve her. One reflexology treatment stopped her headache...five treatments and she was able to go on a week's trip to New York with her family. After coming home, five more treatments were given and she is now WELL and HAPPY. She is back to normal health, and people cannot believe it.

I praise you, Mildred Carter, for your wonderful work. I truly believe in reflexology....It saves lives!

—Ms. L.S.

Children are blessed when they have parents who are caring and concerned for their health. Here is a letter from a mother who used reflexology and saved her teenager's teeth.

Dear Mrs. Carter,

My fourteen-year-old daughter was beginning to have headaches. They were increasing in frequency and severity, and I was wondering if she was under undue stress I wasn't aware of. Meanwhile, I took her to the dentist for a checkup, wondering if there might be something there that would be causing her headaches. Her teeth were fine, but the dentist said her wisdom teeth were crowding her mouth and needed to come out. He wanted to put her under a general anesthetic and *pull all four at once.* My daughter said, "I bet that's what is causing my headaches, Mom." I said, "Wait a minute; let me think this over at home.

I went home and massaged her feet. There was *not even* the *slightest* tenderness in the area of the reflex to the teeth and jaw. But I did find extreme soreness in the neck area and spine. After several trips to the chiropractor, who confirmed my suspicions, and a second opinion from another dentist, my daughter still has her wisdom teeth, but *no more headaches*!

—C.E.

In October I received a letter from a very concerned mother regarding her baby's ear infection. She said that her baby was going to have surgery on her eardrum to stop infections. The mother wanted to use reflexology to treat her little girl. She felt with God's help, she would cure the ear infections.

In December, I received this note from her:

Dear Mrs. Carter,

I offer my THANKS to you, Mildred, for teaching me this wonderful method of reflexology. My baby does NOT need to have surgery for any ear problems. I use reflexology on my baby regularly for maintenance of her good health.

—P.S.L.E.

One of the most exciting and satisfying experiences in life is that of parenthood. Take time for your children; don't let a day go by that you don't listen and talk with your child. Give them all the love you can, and this will help them become well adjusted, secure individuals, and know a more positive world.

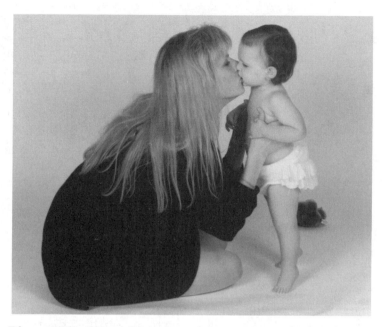

Photo "K": Give children lots of sincere, unconditional love.

CHAPTER 36

How to Use Special Reflexology Devices to Relieve Pain

Dr. Wm. H. Fitzgerald, founder of Zone Therapy, made use of several devices found in the kitchen to help him hold a steady pressure on the reflex buttons for a long period of time. In cases of toothache, earache, labor pains, painful back, and many other painful ailments, he found he could deaden the part of the body to which the reflex went. To save time and to enable his patients to treat themselves at home, Dr. Fitzgerald showed them how to use such common devices as rubber bands, rubber balls, clothespins, and combs.

Reflexology is a natural way to health, and it is not essential that you have reflex devices to obtain benefits. The natural use of your fingers will work wonders in releasing the universal flow of the vital force and sending it surging through all the channels of your body. However, rubber bands, a comb, or another such device can be helpful in putting steady pressure on reflex buttons.

During my years of giving reflexology treatments, I devised several improvements over such old-fashioned implements. You can see my reflexology devices in use in several of the illustrations. You can use these devices safely in your home, your office, or while traveling. If for some reason you cannot find the reflex devices I describe here in your local health food or drugstore, they are available at Stirling Enterprises, Inc., Box 216, Cottage Grove, Oregon 97424.

You will often need assistance in reaching many of the reflexes, both for massaging and for holding a steady pressure on many locations. My reflex massagers enable you to get this help.

REFLEX FOOT MASSAGER

Look at the reflex foot massager. It is simple to use, yet packs a healing power that you will never want to be without. Just place the massager on the floor; using it on a rug will keep it from slipping. Place both of your feet on the ridges of the massager and roll them back and forth. You will find you can massage most of the reflexes in your feet this way. After some practice, you will be able to use these ridges to massage along the reflexes to the spine, the eyes, and so on. There are raised buttons in the center of the reflex massager which will help reach into certain deeper, hard-to-reach reflexes in the feet. See Photos 42 and 43.

If you spend time in front of the TV, this reflex foot massager is invaluable. Just sit back and relax, place your feet on this magic reflex roller, and massage away all your aches and pains. *Don't use it for very long at first.* You will probably find yourself more relaxed than you have felt in years. Many people report that they never knew what a good night's sleep was until they started using reflexology. Remember, you are helping nature rejuvenate the entire body—naturally.

The Purpose of the Pressure

The purpose in using reflex pressure is to release local contraction of muscles and blood vessels or constriction of other soft tissues. Reflexology breaks a vicious cycle occurring in local short-circuited nerves. A reflexology treatment improves lymphatic drainage and steps up your blood supply. It releases waste products that have collected in local areas in amounts sufficient to cause discomfort and pain.

REFLEX ROLLER MASSAGER

Let us now look at the reflex roller massager. This is being used throughout the world by many grateful people. This beautiful little roller will search out every tender reflex button in your body. You can use it to roll over the bottoms of your feet and on your ankles, for your gonads. You can run the little roller up your leg close to the calf, move it over, and run it up the leg closer to the bone to the knee, and under and around the knee, all the time searching for tender reflex spots. It will be hard for you to realize that you could have so many tender spots in your body. Use this reflex roller on the outside of your leg also, up the thigh on the outside, rolling it in many places on the leg, holding a light pressure. When you come to a tender button, run the roller back and forth over the button or, having found the spot that needs to be stimulated with the universal life force, press and massage it with your fingers for a few seconds.

You may use this little magic roller anywhere on your body. It is great to have a partner massage the back, up and down each side of the spine. Do not massage directly on the spine with the roller or any device that you might have. A light pressure on certain vertebrae where directed is okay.

Look at the illustrations of the various uses of this reflex roller. See Photos 6, 7, 29, 31, 34, 41, 44, and 63. Remember, you heal the whole body by opening up closed electrical lines to allow the universal life force to flow freely. You will be amazed at the phenomenal results that you will get from using this roller massager to help you find all the buttons leading to blockage of the energy field.

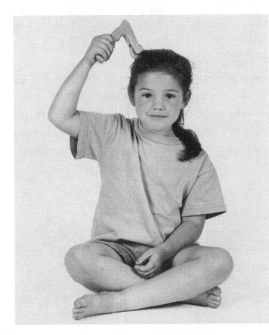

Photo 63: Let us start early in teaching our children the natural way to health through the use of reflexology.

REFLEX HAND PROBE

Now, let us look at the fantastic little reflex hand probe that is being used throughout the world. It takes the place of your fingers and keeps them from becoming tired. Many people's hands are too weak to press the reflex buttons properly. Their fingers get tired, so they turn to this handy little reflex hand probe. It can be used on any reflex in the body where your fingers would otherwise massage. Photos 28, 33, 35, and 64 show this fantastic little hand probe being used.

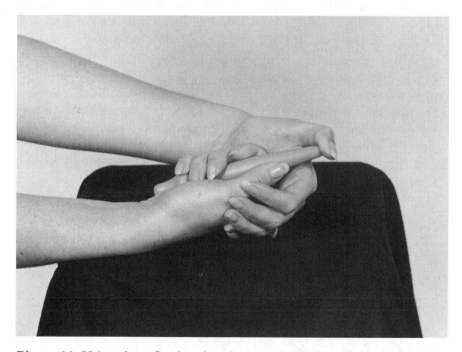

Photo 64: Using the reflex hand probe to massage the reflexes in the thumb to stimulate the pineal and pituitary glands.

Many people tell me that they have used a pencil, but a pencil is hard to hold and the eraser usually breaks off, so they turn to the reflex hand probe to simplify their reflex treatments. It helps them heal the whole body by opening up closed electrical lines for full circulation of the universal life force to all glands, organs, and cells. This will help you retain complete health throughout your long life.

MAGIC REFLEX MASSAGER

An improvement on a rubber ball, the magic reflex massager presses reflex buttons in the hand when squeezed. See Photo 48. Since developing this device, I have received hundreds of letters from all over the world telling me of the unbelievable results people are getting. They are using this massager to press the reflexes in their hands and stimulate every part of their bodies.

When you begin to use this little massager, start out slowly—do not press with it for over two minutes at a time. It is so powerful in the way it stimulates the reflexes to so many glands at once that to release all this new life force suddenly is a shock. The glands are shocked after they have been almost dormant for a long period of time.

How to Use the Magic Reflex Massager

Take the magic massager in one hand and squeeze your fingers around it. This will make its own little "fingers" press into several reflexes of your hand at once. Roll it over and the massager will press into a different set of reflexes. Each time you roll it a little, it reaches different reflex points. See Photos 32 and 65.

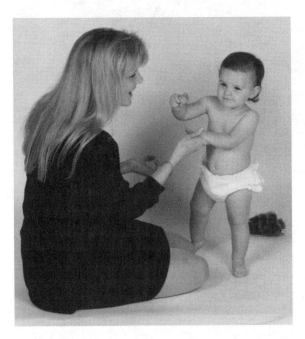

Photo 65: Baby enjoys sterilized magic reflex massager as a toy and as a help in cutting a new tooth.

Roll it in your hand for about two minutes; then change the massager to your other hand, again massaging for about two minutes. You will immediately feel a stimulant of magnetic vitality surging throughout your entire body. You will not want to lay this little magic reflex massager down, but *remember—do not overmassage!* You can pick it up and use it again the next day, or maybe later in the same day. Every individual is different. If your body is in poor condition, use your magic reflex massager for short periods of time at first, with longer periods between massages. Do not try to make yourself completely well in one day.

You can also use the magic reflex massager in both hands at once. Place it in the palm of your left hand. Now cup your right hand over the massager, clasping your fingers around each other. Start rolling your massager in several directions. Feel how the little knobs press into the reflexes of both hands simultaneously. Use this same rolling, pressing motion on your thumbs and on each of your fingers.

The magic reflex massager is helpful in many sports activities. Golfers find that this device provides just the right amount of strength to the muscles needed to swing the club properly. Bowlers find the massager very helpful in keeping their hands and arms strong and relaxed.

Some people use two magic reflex massagers at once, one in each hand, for double benefits. If you look at Diagram 16, you can see how, with two massagers, you can stimulate the reflexes to most of the organs and glands on both sides of your body. By pressing massagers *firmly* with both hands, you will feel tension on every muscle in your body, especially in the inner muscles around your glands and organs.

Reflex exercises for the lower part of your body will not only benefit the lower lumbar area, but also the bladder and urethral channel. They will benefit the reproductive organs to such an extent that many persons feel a renewed interest in sex, as if they have been rejuvenated.

Warning: *Don't overdo this the first week, or you will become very sore and think something has gone wrong with your organs.*

Exercise only once a day for the first two days, then increase to two times a day for two days, and so on, until the muscles have adjusted. This is the same as if you overexercised your legs or arms and got cramps in the muscles. Don't get cramps in the inside muscles. Just take it easy the first week or two, and you will find yourself becoming a new and beautiful you, thanks to the miracles of nature and reflexology.

Tongue Cleaner

For centuries, long before modern mouthwashes came into existence, people in the Orient relied on a natural method for clean, fresh breath—tongue cleaning. You too can use a tongue cleaner to remove odor-causing film deposits. *The tongue cleaner cleans what the toothbrush does not!* In fact, your toothbrush was never intended or designed for your tongue. Use a tongue cleaner after you brush your teeth. Your toothbrush and your tongue cleaner are a perfect combination for superior and complete oral hygiene.

Before you use a tongue cleaner, sterilize it in boiling water for five minutes, or put it in an automatic dishwasher.

Hold the cleaner at both ends, with the middle, curved portion pointing into your mouth. Stretch out your tongue and slowly and gently scrape the upper surface of your tongue with an inside-out motion. See Photo 23. Hold the cleaner under running water to wash off the sticky deposit. Now, you can understand how unclean your tongue was. Repeat the scraping procedure as many times as you feel it is necessary, usually four or five times. Once you get used to cleaning with the tongue cleaner, adjust the scraping pressure to your needs.

At regular intervals, sterilize your tongue cleaner. It is not good hygiene to have more than one person use the same tongue cleaner.

If you are using the tongue cleaner for the first time, your tongue may feel sensitive for a week or so. If this happens, do not be alarmed. No harmful results will occur. Children may use the tongue cleaner, but they should be supervised by an adult.

Palm Massager

The palm massager is a small rubber ball that is still used by many doctors to strengthen the muscles in the arms. It is used in many hospitals to help arthritis sufferers and those overcoming paralysis from various causes.

REFLEX COMB

Pressing and massaging the reflexes with the fingers will give satisfactory results most of the time, but in certain cases a steady pressure will be needed for several minutes at a time. For this, use a comb. You can use any type of comb in an emergency, but keep in mind that most combs are made of plastic. You could very easily break the comb and injure the hands or fingers if too much pressure is placed on the teeth. Therefore, in reflexology, doctors recommend that a metal comb be used. The vibrations of the metal are also thought to help in stimulation of the life forces. Certain metals give off "rays" or "vibrations" that stimulate the current of life forces in the body.

The metal comb is very helpful, for it reaches several reflexes at one time. In Photo 21, you see the tips of the fingers being pressed onto the teeth of the comb while the thumb is pressing on the end of the comb. The teeth of the comb can be used in the webs between the fingers. Also, you can use the back of the comb for a firm, steady pressure.

Other Uses for a Reflex Comb

Take the comb in your hand and press the teeth into the tips of your fingers, pressing your thumb on the end of the comb as shown in Photo 21. If you have two combs, use them both, one in each hand, for a vitalizing sensation of renewed life force.

Try putting the teeth of the comb in different positions. Press the teeth into your first finger on all sides, at the same time pressing your thumb on the end of the comb. This stimulates two important endocrine glands, the pituitary and the pineal. You should feel renewed exhilaration almost instantly. Use this method on all your fingers.

You may also apply the reflex comb effectively on the feet. Press the comb along the pad of your heel to reach all your foot reflexes in this area, working the teeth of the comb down toward your instep, keeping the teeth pressing under your heel pad. Hold pressure on all sore reflexes for a slow count of seven, then release and press again. Repeat this three to five times.

Reflex Clamps

Spring clothespins and rubber bands have been used to press down on reflexes. Reflex clamps, now available, are safer, more comfortable, and easier to use. Many doctors have employed these simple devices to anesthetize various parts of the body and to cure many ailments.

Reflex clamps on the fingers help to relieve pain quickly, and in many cases permanently. Edwin Bowers, M.D., physician and self-helpwriter, states, "This pressure therapy has an advantage over any other method of pain relief, inasmuch as it has been proven that, in contradistinction to opiates, when zone [reflex] pressure relieves pain, it likewise tends to remove the cause of the pain."

In Photo 66 we see that the clamps are on the third, fourth, and fifth fingers of the right hand, stimulating the outer edge of the head and hands and organs on the right side of the body. If the left hand's thumb and second and third fingers are clamped (see Photo 49), we are treating the central part of the left side of the head and corresponding body organs.

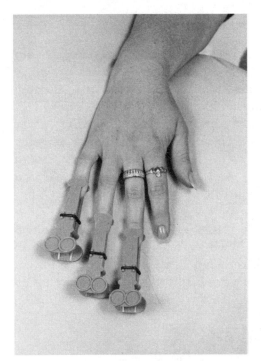

Photo 66: Shows reflex clamp on the third, fourth, and fifth fingers to stimulate or anesthetize the outer part of the head and body.

Reflex clamps keep a steady pressure on the reflex buttons, so you can control several different reflexes at once instead of just one reflex point at a time. This lets you control pain and illnesses faster and more conveniently, especially if you are too ill or in too much pain to press each reflex button with your fingers for any length of time. These clamps may be used on one or several fingers at a time, on your earlobes, or on the webs between the fingers. See Photos 18 and 36. They can also be used on the toes.

Using Reflex Clamps for Vitality

Dear Mrs. Carter,

I cannot tell you how pleased I was at my first use of your reflex clamps. When I put them on my toes, they seemed to stimulate my internal organs and cause my general vigor and vitality to improve by at least 100 percent.

—L.C.

TONGUE DEPRESSOR OR PROBE

A simple tongue depressor solves many health problems. By pressing the reflexes on the tongue, you can stop headaches, toothaches, abdominal pains, menstrual cramps, sore throat, and many other complaints. See Photo 22. It is convenient to carry in your purse and billfold so it can be used in sudden emergencies. *Warning! If you are pregnant, do not use the tongue depressor*; it relaxes the reproductive organs and might cause a miscarriage.

WIRE BRUSH STIMULATES REFLEXES

When you tap the reflexes gently with the metal wires of the brush, you stimulate your electrical life force into immediate action in the area being contacted. The brush is not only great to brush your hair with, but also, when you use it as directed to tap your head and other areas of your body, it can stimulate your whole being into renewed energy and vitality. See Photo 11.

THE MIRACLE OF THE
MINIATURE TRAMPOLINE

Bouncing on a miniature trampoline stresses every cell in your body, over and over again, approximately one hundred times a minute. Every cell is strengthened by this stress. This constant pull and release on all your body cells at the same time helps them become firm and strong.

Henry Savage, M.D., says, "Never in my thirty-five years as a practicing physician have I found any exercise method, at any price, that will do more for the physical body than the rebound exercise."

I know of no more powerful way to build your body into perfect health and keep it that way than by stimulating healthy cell growth with a combination of reflexology and exercising on the rebounder trampoline.

BED RAISERS

Many people raise the foot ends of their beds so they sleep with their heads downward. Thus, for awhile, they reverse the downward pull of gravity on their bodies. The constant daytime downward pull on our bodies is a cause of aging. Body cells become weak and the body tissues begin to sag downward. Even our bones begin to shrink from the constant downward pull of gravity. Thus, you need to get your head lower than your heart at least part of the time. You may lift the foot of your bed either three or six inches to reverse the process of aging.

CHAPTER 37

Reflexology and Your Pets

One of nature's wonders are animals. They are loving uncritical companions, always available for touch and attention, which has been proven to be extremely healing to both our body and soul.

The positive contributions pets make to human health cannot be overlooked. Just the touch of a pet can reduce signs of tension and relieve pain. A pet will take your mind off yourself. Have you ever watched a puppy or kitten play with its tail, or hop on a bag? If so, you probably couldn't help but laugh. Humor has a great influence on sickness, stress, and depression.

The State University College of Veterinary Medicine in Washington has a People-Pet Partnership Program through which the handicapped can go horseback riding. A person who sits in a wheelchair can sit high above all else on a horse, now feeling stronger, bigger, and much happier. There is a bond that builds between animals and people, and for the handicapped, this bond makes life more bearable.

A PET IS THE BEST MEDICINE
FOR A LONELY PERSON

The love of animals plays a big part in many of our lives. To many people, animals take the place of children who have gone from home or children we have never been blessed with. Everyone should have a

pet of some kind. It makes no difference what it is, just so it is something *alive!*

It has been scientifically proven that those suffering from heart
ailments live much longer if they have a pet to love and to keep them
company. A pet is the best medicine for a lonely person, and all pets
are quite intelligent, no matter what they are. Even though some have
tiny brains, they surprise you with their response to your love and care.
I have had just about every kind of pet that you could think of, and
there was not one of them that I could not relate to—even a spider
that my patient mother let me keep in the kitchen for a long time when
I didn't have a pet to love. Science is now proving that all life has great
intelligence, so why wouldn't they respond to our loving care.

How Reflexology Can Help Your Animal

When your animal becomes ill, try reflexology. Use the same methods as described in this book for people. Search for tender areas all
over the body, especially on the pads of the feet. When the animal
flinches, this means you have found a reflex to a malfunctioning
gland or organ or to an injury some place in the body. Just press and
roll your finger or thumb on the tender button as much as the animal will let you. They seem to understand what you are trying to do
and will willingly let you carry on the reflex work, even if it is
painful. However, if a sick animal does not appear friendly, respect
his wishes and leave him rest.

Of course when first introducing your animal to reflexology, go
slowly. It may help to start rubbing gently on areas you know he
enjoys, such as favorite spots around the head, cheeks, under the chin
and on the neck, back and tail (and in addition, for dogs, their stomach and groin.) When your animal is relaxed and knows he can trust
you, take the foreleg and work with slow and gentle pressure, both on
top and bottom of the foot. Work reflexes between each pad, then roll
each toe between your index finger and thumb a few times. Work the
tendons and reflexes up the leg. You will want to support the leg with
one hand, as you work with the other. Work on up and around the
entire foreleg, work across the attaching tendons and muscles, pay
special attention at wrist (near the dewclaw) and elbow joints. Be gentle. Repeat on hind foot and leg.

Now using both of your hands, grasp your animal gently by all four legs and turn it over onto its other side. Again start with the foot on the foreleg and work up. Repeat procedure on rear leg, all the way to the base of tail. Work each area with a pressing circular motion.

You can work reflexes on other parts of your animals in the same way. Remember you are actually working the reflexes below the skin, so do not rub the skin surface. Relax your animal by holding your fingertips together and working them in little circles down alongside the spine. (Do not press on the vertebrae themselves.) If you see your animal flinch when you press certain points, go easier, as it may be a very tender point.

When you know that there is a specific condition that seems to be throwing the animal's body system out of order, all you have to do is to work the corresponding reflex to release a free flow of life energy back into the malfunctioning area. If you work on an area that seems to be especially sensitive or tender, or if the animal seems to have a weak limb, just rub your hands together and place them over the area for a minute, letting warmth and energy penetrate. You can talk to the animal and encourage it to get well and tell it to heal perfectly.

Pets are a luxury! They depend solely on you for their existence. So be good to them...they deserve a good life.

A Nice Finishing Touch

When you have completed the reflex session, it is a nice finishing touch to pet your animal, from head to toes. You can start on the side that is already facing upward. Pet gently along the top of the head, along the neck, all the way down the back to the hip, then on down the back leg to the paw. Now go back to the shoulder of the foreleg and pet down to the paw. Slowly stroke and pet with one or both of your hands five times. You can turn your animal over and pet the other side in the same way. Your pet will be very relaxed.

I get many letters from people who have used reflexology to help their pets overcome illnesses their veterinarians were not able to cure. In many cases, the animals guide their owners to the very reflexes that need stimulation by biting or scratching certain areas. Mr. J. wrote me to tell of his success in healing his valuable watch dog of an unknown illness.

Valuable Watchdog Healed

Dear Mrs. Carter,

Borax is a Great Dane dog, six years old. He has always been very healthy, up until a month ago. He is a very important guard dog for our business, besides a loving companion for my whole family.

One morning, when I went into the yard, Borax did not come to greet me as usual. I found him lying in his bed very ill and shaking all over.

I rushed him to the veterinarian and after a careful examination, the vet could not find anything the matter with him so they wanted to do an exploratory operation. I refused and carried Borax home to give nature a chance to heal him.

The vet said that sometimes animals have their own cures if left alone. The dog was ill for several days but didn't seem to get any better or any worse; he just lay quietly in his bed. I started to watch him, and I noticed that on several occasions, he would get up and try to scratch his back on the top of his doghouse. So I thought of reflexology and the things you had said about animals in your wonderful book. I started to feel along Borax's back for tender spots. I ran my hands with pressure all along both sides of the back and down the sides, feeling for a tender reflex button. He seemed to understand what I was doing and kept turning around, turning his right side to me. I concentrated on that side and sure enough, I came across a spot that made him flinch and cry out. I knew that I had found the cause of his trouble. I worked the area very gently, at first; as the pain subsided, I worked it harder.

I used this pressing and rolling technique with my fingers on him several times that day, and by evening, he was able to stand up and wag his tail and take food. In two days, he was back to his old happy self, romping and playing with the children. We never knew what Borax's problem was, but I am sure that he would have died if we hadn't used reflexology on him. We all feel that you are responsible for saving the life of our greatly loved companion and no words can thank you enough!

Thanks and God bless,

—Mr. J.

Dear Mrs. Carter,

I want to tell you about my little dog and reflexology. I noticed that he was licking and biting at his left foot almost constantly, so I thought I'd better examine it and see what was wrong.

I couldn't find anything the matter with the foot. I examined the toes, foot, and leg, but on further investigation, I discovered the cat had scratched his eye, and he had a big nick out of his eye.

I took him to the vet, who gave me some drops to put in the eye to heal it. But my dog continued to lick and bite his foot on the same side on which the eye was injured. After that, I worked the reflexes on his foot several times, and his eye was soon healed.

To me, this proves that animals instinctively turn to reflexology to heal their ailments. It might be wise to check your pet when you see him licking and biting at his feet. He may be trying to heal a problem elsewhere in the body.

Thank you, and God bless you for reflexology.

Sincerely,

—Mrs. J.W.

Dear Mrs. Carter,

I feel I know you through your video and books! Just a note to tell you how reflexology helped our family member, Roger. He is a beautiful golden retriever and was starting to have symptoms of old age. He seemed to sleep most of the time and showed signs of stiffness in his rear joints. His general appearance was dull.

We used a basic reflexology workout on his paws, once a day. We worked on each paw for approximately one minute, then would work on another one. The whole session only lasted about five minutes. We also added one teaspoon of brewer's yeast in his food and gave him a bone meal tablet once a day. Roger is now jogging with us again and his signs of stiffness seem to be gone. It is good to have him back as an "active" member of our family.

Thanks a million for your great teachings.

—T.G.

Reflexology Helps AKS Champion

Dear Mrs. Carter,

With guidance and a lot of T.L.C. my puppy became a champion show dog. When she had puppies, my friend kept one. Again with perseverance we trained the puppy, Muffin, and it also became a champion. Muffin, now fifteen years old, was introduced to reflexology last week. My friend was so pleased that she made appointments twice weekly for the two of them to have reflexology workouts.

—P.C.

So when your pet is feeling out of sorts, turn to reflexology to promote better circulation, relaxation, and health. Regular sessions will strengthen the affectionate bond between you and your pet. Pets are our companions, and they bring comfort through touch. No person with a pet is without a family.

Conclusion: Heal Thyself and Thy Neighbor

In this book, I have given you several natural methods of healing from the very simplest headache to the most serious of chronic degenerative diseases.

I have not written this book for you to read and cast aside. I want you to put it to daily use for yourself, your loved ones, and your neighbors.

I have devoted my life to research so that I might be able to bring every man, woman, child, and even animal a natural, simple, harmless way to live a life free from pain and illness, safe and free! I want you to understand and learn to use God's most precious gift, *reflexology*, nature's way to perfect health.

It would be impossible for me to reveal in one book all the miraculous methods of natural healing that I have discovered in my many years of research throughout the world.

I can truthfully say that in all my traveling and research, here and abroad, I have never found any method of healing that can compare with the simple dynamic healing power of reflexology.

Although I have given you a few other methods of natural healing to use along with reflexology, I want you to know that reflexology is the primary key to natural healing of every illness and freedom from pain when used as directed.

Although this book deals mostly with physical and material aspects of gaining health and freedom from pain, keep in mind that the real purpose of attaining a healthy, long life is to recognize the higher divine purpose for which we were born. Perfect health would be wasted unless the healthy body is used as a temple for our spirit to

331

develop in. Our life on this planet is a schooling period to enable us to improve and perfect our human and divine characteristics.

Through the directions given in this book and my previous books on foot and hand reflexology, you may use this dynamic power of natural healing for yourself and for those who are crying out in anguished suffering and despair—by the simple method of pressing certain electrical reflex buttons located throughout the body. Although different bodies require different medication and vitamins, *reflexology works the same for all bodies.*

I have given you the key to the source and the power to heal. Open the door, step in, and heal thy neighbor and thyself.

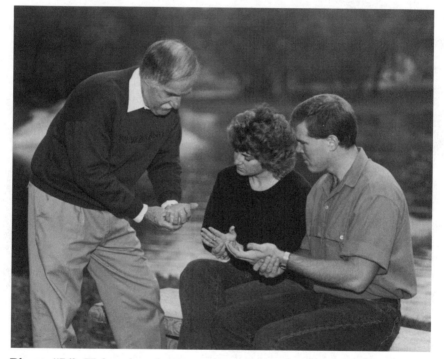

Photo "L": Help others learn to promote renewed health, vigor and youthfulness.

Index

If you are interested in purchasing any of the reflexology devices shown in this book, you may send $2.00 for a catalog, which will be refunded on your first order.

Write to: **STIRLING ENTERPRISES, INC.**
           P. O. BOX 216
           COTTAGE GROVE, OREGON 97424

Or call 1–503–942–4622.

Phone ordering hours:
Monday through Thursday 9:00 A.M. – 3:00 P.M. Pacific Time.

Remember: Catalog Shopping saves you time and gas looking for these unique products.

"Dear Ms. Carter,

I want to tell you how grateful I am for your wonderful books. I speak about your books to everyone that I know or meet and I have great faith in reflexology. I hope to see the day when operations, drugs and medicines of all sorts will vanish, thus leave room for the natural God-given way to gain back good health and keep our health naturally.

Thanks again. May God Bless you."

—M.R., Canada

"Dear Ms. Carter,

First, I would like to tell you that your book, *Helping Yourself with Foot Reflexology*, is one of the most important possessions we have.

We are three generations who are artists but we live on two hundred forty acres on a homestead farm in northern Minnesota. We came here eight years ago and have a pottery business and do organic gardening. Your book has saved many a doctor bill. Doctors are notoriously bad here, and we are grateful to you. We live in the boonies on a dirt road, so in winters (though we do get out most of the time) we count on your book and organic foods from our garden to keep us going. I don't know what we would do without the information of using reflexology. Thank you for your great book and all the help you have given us.

Very sincerely yours,"

—B.W.P., U.S.A.

"Dear Mrs. Carter,

I work with a group of men who travel to wherever our jobs take us. We do not have medical aid or doctors in some of the locations we have been sent to. We each learned to be our own best doctor when there was none available. We use your books to guide us with our health. Reflexology has helped us in many ways, for many years."

—C.V. and Team

"Dear Ms. Carter,

Having read your book, *Helping Yourself with Foot Reflexology*, I wish to learn more about it. I have the opportunity to come to the U.S.A. in July, and I would be interested in any kind of training program in reflexology you could recommend to me.

Thank you. I am grateful for the learning about reflexology. I hope I will have the opportunity to learn more.

Yours sincerely,"

—R. P.

"Dear Ms. Carter,

First of all, I am deeply grateful for your wonderful book, *Hand Reflexology, Key to Perfect Health,* which is helping me and my friends very much. I know that you are receiving thousands of letters from all over the world with the same expression of gratitude. Nevertheless, I can't help but do the same, for I feel the need to tell you personally what joy, truly, you have given me and my friends. God reward you a millionfold.

I repeat, you have done a wonderful work—a lifetime legacy to the whole world. Congratulations, and I thank you without end. I hope to hear from you. Keeping you in our prayers, I remain,"

—L.M.T., Carmelite Monastery